Health and Ways of Living

HEALTH AND WAYS OF LIVING

The Alameda County Study

LISA F. BERKMAN, Ph.D.
Associate Professor of Epidemiology and Public Health
Yale University

LESTER BRESLOW, M.D., M.P.H.
Professor of Public Health
University of California, Los Angeles

New York   Oxford
OXFORD UNIVERSITY PRESS
1983

Library of Congress Cataloging in Publication Data
Berkman, Lisa F.
Health and ways of living.
Bibliography: p.   Includes index.
1. Health behavior.   2. Diseases—Causes and theories of causation.
3. Health behavior—California—Alameda County.
4. Health status indicators—California—Alameda County.
5. Health surveys—California—Alameda County.
6. Alameda County (Calif.)—Statistics, Medical.
I. Breslow, Lester.   II. Title [DNLM: 1. Life style.
2. Health surveys—California. WA 900 AC2 B5h]
RA776.9.B47   1983   616.07′1   82-7941

Printing (last digit): 9 8 7 6 5 4 3 2 1

Printed in the United States of America

To
JOSEPH HOCHSTIM
and
ANDREI and ALEXANDER

Preface

This book has grown over a long period of time with the help of several people. Preliminary work on the health practices was first published over a decade ago by Nedra Belloc and Lester Breslow. The analyses of social networks were first done by Lisa Berkman for her dissertation in 1977. Much of the methodological work included in Chapter 2 was done by Joseph Hochstim in the late 1960's and early 1970's. We thought it would be very useful to bring all this information together and combine it with the most recent follow-up of the Alameda County cohort.

In looking at the present analyses of the cohort first surveyed in 1965 and subsequently followed through 1974, we have been struck by the consistency and similarity of our findings. Most of the factors of interest to us seemed to have very broad health consequences. And in most cases, these effects were evident in the 1965 health assessments, the nine-year mortality risks, and the changes in health status occurring between 1965 and 1974.

To give the reader some feeling of just how broad the health consequences of health practices and social networks are, we have presented findings concerning both mortality and changes in self-reported health status. The first chapter of the book gives the reader our perspectives on changes in health that have occurred over the last century and an overview of critical issues in the field. The second chapter supplies background information on the Human Population Laboratory including the purposes of the HPL, sampling methods, response rates, and validity and reliability of survey items.

The relationship of health practices with mortality risk is the topic of Chapter 3; data are presented for each practice individually as well as in a cumulative index. Chapter 4 describes the association between social networks and mortality risk. Again, each type of social contact is analyzed individually as well as in a cumulative Social Network Index. In both these chapters the effects of physical health status and socioeconomic status are examined in detail. Chapter 5 is a multivariate analysis of the health practices and social networks in which the effects of many variables on mortality risk are considered simultaneously. In Chapter 6, Camacho and Wiley study the changes in physical health status that occurred in the interval between the two study periods, 1965–1974, and assess the effects of health practices and social networks on such changes.

The final chapter is a discussion and summary of the findings presented in Chapters 3 through 6. Thus, we have approached the study of health and ways of living from many angles. In some cases, the questions on a certain topic, while adequate in 1965, do not meet the most sophisticated standards in existence now. We hope, however, that we have exploited the data set to its fullest and that this book will serve to spur new interest in the effects of common health-related behaviors and social conditions on health status.

Acknowledgments

When a study is over twenty years old, there are a lot of people to thank. First, we would like to acknowledge our debt to the 6928 men and women of Alameda County who participated in our survey. Respondents often go unacknowledged, and while they receive little personal benefit from filling out our questionnaires and being tracked down wherever their lives may lead them over the ensuing decades, they are the cornerstone of all epidemiologic research. They have contributed substantially to our understanding of health and ways of living, and we thank them. Hopefully, this book will repay them, in some small part, for the time they have given us over the years.

Secondly, this study has been funded since its inception by the National Center for Health Services Research. Funding for such broadly based health surveys is hard to come by, and the extended and steady support of NCHSR has been greatly appreciated. We would like to thank two individuals at NCHSR for their particular interest in the Human Population

Laboratory: William Lohr and Ralph Sloat have always been very helpful to us, even in difficult times. The HPL was supported by NCHSR Grant No. HS00368. The HPL has also always been part of the California Department of Health Services. Thanks go to them for supporting our research efforts in many different ways.

In addition to the authors of various chapters of this book, many individuals have participated significantly in the Human Population Laboratory over the years. We particularly want to acknowledge the contributions of four persons who have been instrumental in the conceptual and epidemiologic aspects of the Human Population Laboratory: Joseph Hochstim, Ira Cisin, Dimitri Athanasopolous, and John Finan. Four other people have made outstanding contributions to the conduct of operations and data analysis: Allen Carrington, Nedra Belloc, Paul Berkman, and George Kaplan. It is no exaggeration to say that this study would never have been completed without the enormous efforts of Allen Carrington who throughout the years has been responsible for the ongoing administration of the project and the tracing and follow-up of almost 7000 respondents. We thank him. Nedra Belloc and Paul Berkman provided critical insights into the data. Their thoughts and ideas have influenced the course of the study. George Kaplan is the project's current director and the course he is steering now is again an exciting one. The work of these eight people made possible the studies reported here.

Ideas for studies such as this one are not created in a vacuum. We would like to thank several of our colleagues for their valuable intellectual support and insights. The thoughts of S. Leonard Syme are sprinkled throughout this volume as are the ideas of Aaron Antonovsky and John Cassel. The early epidemiologic work of Wade Hampton Frost and John Sydenstricker have been powerful influences on our work. Our colleagues at the Human Population Laboratory at the time when much of the book was written have been enormously helpful to us: Jim Wiley, Deborah Wingard, Terry Camacho, and, again, Allen Carrington. Many days were spent discussing issues explored in the monograph. Special thanks go to Wanda Nicoletti for typing the first copies of the manuscript and to Elizabeth Mailloux at Yale for typing the many revisions which followed. Sincere thanks must be extended to our editor at Oxford, Jeffrey House. He has been an especially resourceful and tactful writer, editor, and sometime arbitrator.

Having acknowledged the financial and intellectual support of our friends and colleagues, we would like to acknowledge the emotional support provided by our spouses, Miklos Pogany and Devra Breslow. Writing a book is at least as hard on spouses as it is on authors.

I, (L. F. B.) would like to extend special thanks to my parents Anne and Stuart Berkman for always supporting and encouraging my desire to work. Finally, this book has spanned the births of two children, Andrei and Alexander Pogany, one of whom is now old enough to tell his mother to have a good day at work and write a chapter! Thanks.

New Haven, Connecticut   L. F. B.
July 1983   L. B.

Contents

Health and Ways of Living

1. Introduction and background

Research as well as common sense indicates that the way people live, what they do day after day, profoundly affects their health. Investigators are finding that the social environment and certain common behaviors such as physical activity, use of alcohol and tobacco, and eating and sleeping habits are related to the major diseases of our time. Industrialization and urbanization demand less physical exertion of individuals, promote extensive dietary changes, and change social and work patterns, and this has evidently created a new set of health problems. In the developed world, these conditions have replaced the gross insanitation, overcrowding, undernutrition, and physical exhaustion of the nineteenth century as major determinants of health.

The idea that ways of living are related to health is not new. In the Western World, the Greeks and Romans recognized the importance of preventing illness through living sensibly. Hygeia, the Greek goddess of health, represented the view that "health is the natural order of things, and a positive attribute to which men are entitled if they govern their lives wisely" (Dubos, 1959). Medicine's most important function, according to this viewpoint, was to discover the natural laws by which human beings were ensured "a healthy mind in a healthy body." The idea of host susceptibility to illness was part of classical medical thought (Hippocrates, 1938; Sigerist, 1933; Stewart, 1968), and the philosophy of maintaining health by living properly has roots not only in Western, but also in Chinese, Middle Eastern, and other ancient civilizations.

The purpose of this monograph is to explore the relationship between certain behaviors and social connections of individuals—ways of living and physical health status—and mortality. In our exploration of these relationships, we have been guided by two thoughts. The first is that in most industrialized countries new living circumstances are responsible for an increasingly large proportion of the morbidity and mortality among middle-aged and older adults. These disease determinants reside primarily within the social environment and promote certain distinctive behaviors. They have always been related to health status in some way, but may previously have been obscured by other causative factors including exposure to virulent and infectious organisms.

The second thought concerns the precise role these social and behavioral factors play in causing disease. Most epidemiologic investigations, and medical research in general, focus on the relationship between specific factors and specific diseases. It is becoming increasingly apparent, however, that some factors are associated with a wide range of diseases and may, in fact, influence susceptibility to disease in general. Social and behavioral factors appear to be particularly likely to influence health status in this way. Thus our investigation concentrates on sets of these factors that may be associated with many diseases.

Scientific thinking has been slowly heading in this direction. In this chapter we will trace the developments that led to this study, but emphasize at the outset that this brief excursion will outline only certain major events. For readers interested in a more thorough examination of medical history and trends in disease distribution, references cited will provide greater detail.

In the nineteenth century, the Industrial Revolution spread through Europe and North America, drawing people from the countryside into cities to work in new factories. The cities, which grew rapidly, were not well equipped to deal with the problems engendered by the rapid influx of people. Gross sewage pollution of water supplies caused outbreaks of water-borne infectious diseases, primarily cholera, dysentery, and typhoid fever. Crowding, poor housing, inadequate nutrition, and exhausting working conditions aggravated water-borne diseases and promoted air-borne diseases such as tuberculosis, bronchitis, whooping cough, measles, diphtheria, scarlet fever, and smallpox (Frost, 1941; McKeown, 1976; Rosen, 1975). These communicable diseases posed severe health threats to urban populations and thus held back industrial growth. Efforts to control them became critical.

The factors that were eventually responsible for curtailing infectious disease in industrialized countries had several origins. Perhaps the most widely recognized were the sciences of pathology and bacteriology, whose development was stimulated by the dominance of infectious disease in the nineteenth century. Another contributing science was epidemiology, whose early findings pointed toward environmental control of infectious disease. Improvements in economic conditions that raised the standard of living in the nineteenth and early twentieth century also promoted health.

The germ theory: disease specificity

The major contributions of bacteriology and pathology were to isolate microorganisms that caused specific diseases and to define their characteristic features. These advances resulted both from technological progress in the sciences and from an improved understanding of disease causation, including specific criteria that linked a specific organism to a specific disease. The set of postulates formulated by Koch (1890) and Henle (1933) has been discussed in detail by many authors (Evans, 1976; Stewart, 1968; Susser, 1973). Briefly, they require that the pathogen must meet the following conditions:

1. Invariably associated with a given disease
2. Isolated in pure culture from the characteristic lesion of the disease
3. Able to reproduce the disease
4. Reisolated in pure culture from the lesion

For our purposes, it is important to know that this set of postulates, along with the germ theory of disease that was developed in the mid-nineteenth century, gave rise to the view that illness consisted of many discrete clinical entities, each caused by a different agent (such as a bacterium), and each with certain morbid manifestations yielding distinct syndromes. This view gained ascendancy as bacteriologists pinpointed specific microorganisms as the cause of condition after condition. The idea of disease specificity took strong root. It appeared that the future of health progress lay in differentiating diseases, discovering their specific causes (principally microorganisms), and then preventing these agents from being carried by vectors to human hosts.

This general approach later incorporated the idea of other discrete causes of specific diseases such as viruses, toxic substances, and vitamin deficiencies. Medical science pursued vigorously the one disease–one cause model.

Susceptibility to illness was similarly regarded as highly specific. Susceptibility to diphtheria, for example, was attributed to the lack of certain antibodies against the causative organism. Resistance in the form of these antibodies could be acquired by natural exposure to the diphtheria bacilli,

by injection of antibodies produced in the blood serum of animals delib-
erately exposed to the organism, for temporary effect, or by injection of
antibody-stimulating antigen made from organisms, for active and lasting
immunity. Along the lines of this bacterial approach, disease after disease
was attacked by attempting to avoid or destroy specific causative agents,
or to develop resistance to them. Bacteriology set the pace not only for
medicine but for health work in general.

Evans (1976) noted that although Koch's postulates have been rigidly
regarded by many scientists as the only true basis for establishing disease
causation, Koch himself understood that there were limitations to the
postulates and that an agent might cause disease without fulfilling all the
criteria. Moreover, many practitioners of medicine who were Koch's
contemporaries waged a battle against the "germ theory" of the bacteriologists; however, they were soon overwhelmed by the proponents of the
new theory. As Dubos (1965) pointed out:

These vague arguments were no match for the precise experimentation by which
Pasteur, Koch, and their followers defended the doctrine of specific causation of
disease. Experimental science triumphed over the clinical art, and within a decade
the theory of specific etiology of disease was all but universally accepted, soon
becoming, as we have seen, the dominant force in medicine.

There is no doubt that the germ theory approach expedited the identification of discrete exogenous agents capable of causing many diseases. A
model of disease causation, however, that relies exclusively on finding
single agents as the sufficient and necessary causes of specific disease has
certain limitations that impair the understanding of disease rates during
the last 150 years.

In tracing the history of understanding disease causation, Evans (1976)
revealed the difficulties that infectious disease researchers encountered in
trying to fulfill Koch's criteria for determining etiology. A causative link
between infectious mononucleosis and Epstein-Barr virus, for instance,
was established without fulfilling a single one of Koch's postulates (Henle
et al., 1968). Similarly, Koch's postulates could not be fulfilled in finding
the causative relationship of slow viruses to such diseases as Kuru and
Creutzfeldt-Jakob disease (Gajdusek, 1973). These examples may seem
merely rare exceptions to the general rule. It should be noted, however,
that many viruses and bacteria known to be pathogenic are present in
people showing no clinical symptoms of disease. Even in the case of acute
infectious diseases, the causes of which are most likely to be illuminated
by Koch's postulates, it appears that the infectious agent is a necessary,
but not usually a sufficient, factor in their etiology. As Evans (1976)

stated, "co-factors and the susceptibility of the host (are) of key importance in the occurrence of clinical illness."

An impressive decline in infectious disease morbidity and mortality has
certainly occurred in industrialized countries over the last century and a
half. How much the germ theory contributed to this decline is not as clear,
however, as it may appear. On one hand, with Koch's postulates germ
theorists did make notable discoveries. Adoption of public health measures based on their findings did prevent the transmission of microorganisms via particular vectors to a host. Human excrement, no matter how
dilute, was kept out of water supplies. Efforts were made to eliminate
living disease organisms from water, milk, and other food supplies by
pasteurization of milk and improved sanitation procedures for food and
water. Semmelweis (1941) instituted hospital procedures that prevented
physicians and medical students from transmitting infectious material
from ward to ward. Lister, in order to combat "atmospheric germs," introduced new surgical procedures based on sanitary principles (Sigerist, 1933).

There is little doubt that these environmental interventions led to a
decrease in infectious disease rates. It is also important to note, however,
that epidemiologic evidence indicated associations between certain factors
and diseases, and that evidence led to successful public health measures
before the actual microorganisms responsible for the disease were identified. For example, a decade before Pasteur initiated the bacteriology era
and three decades before Koch discovered the cholera vibrio, John Snow
showed that cholera was transmitted by fecal-contaminated water and
could be curtailed by eliminating such contamination (Snow, 1936).

Many of these environmental interventions had broader effects than
originally anticipated. For instance, pasteurizing milk and supervising
catttle and milk supplies, primarily in an effort to contain tuberculosis,
also destroyed other harmful agents (Krause, 1928). Many of these agents
caused severe diarrheal disease and were associated with high infant
mortality rates. Other efforts to control tuberculosis among factory
workers seemed to reinforce social movements to improve conditions in
factories and workshops (Linenthal, 1908). Rosen (1975) referred to such
consequences as "synergistic preventive efforts" or "broad-spectrum prevention."

The decline in infectious disease rates is commonly attributed to medical interventions based on concepts of disease specificity in which antibiotics, other chemotherapeutic agents, and immunizations are given to
individuals. It is evident, though, that broad environmental measures have
contributed substantially to disease control. Analyses of time trends reveal
that mortality rates from individual infectious diseases, as well as from all

causes, had been falling since the middle of the nineteenth century in industrializing countries. Such declines antedate the introduction of antibiotics and, in most cases, immunization programs (Dubos, 1959; McKeown, 1976; Porter, 1972). Public health efforts, and particularly changes in social and environmental conditions, were more influential than specific medical intervention.

Tuberculosis, a major cause of death in the nineteenth and early twentieth centuries, has consistently and steadily declined since at least the mid-nineteenth century in many industrialized countries. Clearly, significant declines started to occur well before drug therapy or other therapeutic procedures were available to large populations (McKeown, 1976; Powles, 1973). McKeown has estimated the amount of decline in tuberculosis death rates that can be attributed to the introduction of chemotherapy in England and Wales. His calculations indicate that whereas the death rate from tuberculosis fell by one-half during the quarter century after streptomycin became available (1948–1971), for the total period since tuberculosis deaths were first recorded (1848–1971) the reduction was only 3.2 percent (see Figure 1-1).

In the United States, by 1900, tuberculosis had retreated to second place among the causes of death. From 1900 on, the tuberculosis death rate declined steadily and was only accelerated with the introduction of chemotherapy. Wade Hampton Frost, a noted epidemiologist who studied the decline in tuberculosis mortality, observed in 1937 before the introduction of effective chemotherapy:

It is probable that one of the most important factors in the decline in tuberculosis has been progressively increasing human resistance, due to the influence of selective mortality and to environmental improvements, such as better nutrition and relief from physical stress tending to raise what may be called nonspecific resistance.

Rosen (1975) suggested that the decline in tuberculosis morbidity and mortality could be seen as an expression of an evolving biosocial process involving biologic characteristics of the tubercle bacillus, characteristics of the human host, and environmental factors in a dynamic equilibrium.

Diphtheria has been accurately diagnosed by bacteriologic methods and treated effectively with antitoxin since the nineteenth century. By the turn of the century mass immunization programs among schoolchildren were initiated in the United States (Park et al., 1923; Zingher, 1921). Although the conquering of diphtheria was undoubtedly largely a result of mass immunization programs, some findings indicate that other factors must have played a role. Foremost is the observation that the decline actually started in the nineteenth century before diphtheria antitoxin was

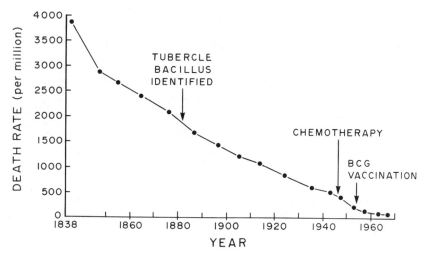

Fig. 1-1. Respiratory tuberculosis: mean annual death rates (standardized to 1901 population) in England and Wales. (*From* McKeown, T.: *The Role of Medicine: Dream, Mirage or Nemesis?* London: Nuffield Provincial Hospital Trust, 1976, p. 81.)

generally used (Rosen, 1975). In 1894 in New York City the death rate among children up to 10 years of age was 785 per 100,000. By 1900, it had fallen below 300 per 100,000. An epidemic wave may decline for many reasons. It is clear, however, that medical intervention did not significantly influence the large early decline of tuberculosis and diphtheria.

A review of mortality rates from infectious diseases in Sweden reveals that for only 3 of 13 diseases studied did the introduction of drugs accelerate the decline in mortality (Hemminki and Paakkulainen, 1976).

These data indicate that immunization and chemotherapeutic interventions may not have played the singularly critical role in the reduction of morbidity and mortality from infectious disease that is commonly attributed to them. With some notable exceptions, such as poliomyelitis and smallpox, the broad decline in infectious disease rates in industrialized countries seems due, in large part, to other factors. But what are they?

We have already noted the importance of public health interventions involving environmental and sanitary engineering. In addition, other conditions seem to have influenced health status. Substantial social and economic improvements in nutrition, housing, and working conditions in the nineteenth century are well documented (Buer, 1968). McKeown has attributed the decline in many infectious disease rates to such changing environmental and economic conditions, specifically to better nutrition and living in a more hygienic environment. This notion is supported by the work of Frost on tuberculosis (1941), that of Goldberger, Wheeler, and Sydenstricker on pellagra (1920), and that of many investigators on infant mortality. A decrease in birthrate has also been suggested as an important factor in the improved physical health status of populations during the same time period (McKeown, 1971; Powles, 1973).

If changes in economic and social conditions are related to the improved health status of people in industrialized countries, this relationship is not easily and completely explained by traditional germ theory with its emphasis on etiologic specificity. On the contrary, these changing conditions appear to be associated with very general health outcomes, such as a fall in morbidity and mortality rates from many infectious diseases and a decline in infant and maternal mortality rates. This generalized health outcome may have come about not only because environmental conditions—like water sanitation and less crowding—blocked exposure to a wide variety of specific noxious agents, but also because other simultaneous changes, such as improvements in nutrition and economic status, simply made individuals less vulnerable to disease in general even though they were exposed to particular agents (Newberne and Williams, 1970; Syme and Berkman, 1976). Frost, in his article on control of tuberculosis, noted that environmental improvements promote "nonspecific resistance" to disease (Frost, 1937).

On the basis of the ecologic correlations presented, it seems likely that the decline in infectious disease rates that has occurred in the last 150 years in European and North American countries came about as the result of three sets of factors: (1) the development of the germ theory of disease, which led to disease-specific control efforts; (2) epidemiology and public health measures that led to broad-ranging environmental interventions; and (3) social, economic, and environmental changes that decreased host vulnerability to disease in general and decreased exposure to many noxious agents.

It also seems clear that models of disease causation, even those centered on infectious disease, must represent complex interactions among agent, host, and vector. Understanding causation based solely on Koch's postulates is bound to be limited in significant ways. Evans (1976) outlined the limitations, stating that the postulates:

1. may not be applicable to all pathogenic bacteria;
2. may not be applicable to viruses, fungi, and parasites;
3. do not include concepts of
   (a) the asypmtomatic carrier state,
   (b) the biologic spectrum of disease,
   (c) epidemiologic and immunologic elements of causation,

(d) prevention of disease by elimination of the putative cause as an element of causation,

(e) multiple causation,

(f) the reactivation of latent agents,

(g) the possibility that clinical syndromes have different causes in different settings.

The strengths and limitations of Koch's model are now recognized by most investigators. That model, however, has subtly and extensively penetrated modern epidemiology and has exerted a powerful effect on the methods epidemiologists have used to make causal inferences about diseases. Of particular relevance is the epidemiologic criterion for judging causation termed "specificity of association" (Fox et al. 1972; Lilienfeld, 1980; Mausner and Bahn, 1974). In 1959, Yerushalmy and Palmer stated that the higher the specificity of an observed association, "the higher the validity of the causal inference." Although this is certainly a reasonable statement, some epidemiologists have gone further to suggest that non-specificity casts doubt on any causal relationship. Berkson in the early 1960s (1960, 1962), for instance, argued that neither cigarette smoking nor marital status is etiologically related to disease because these factors are related to so many different disease outcomes. Clearly the evidence linking cigarette smoking causatively to many disease states is now overwhelming, and few would argue against its pervasive effects. The effects of marital status on health status, however, are still widely debated.

In making causal inference, however, epidemiologists tend to use several criteria of which specificity of association is just one. Other common criteria are strength of association, consistency, logical time order, and coherence of association. The inability to fulfill one criterion does not negate the drawing of a causal link between a factor and a disease outcome. Susser (1977) has proposed that "specificity enhances the plausibility of causal inference, but the lack of specificity does not negate it." He and other epidemiologists have argued that there is no logical reason a factor should not have multiple effects and work through a variety of mechanisms. In fact, it has been suggested that some social factors may be causally linked to disease through their effects on physiologic regulatory systems in the body, which are known to increase a person's risk for a set of diseases.

Specificity would seem to be one of several criteria that should be weighed in arriving at a judgment. In practice, however, many epidemiologists still assume that relationships between suspected risk factors and diseases must be specific, and they design studies that reflect that assumption. This attitude has hampered the discovery of factors that have general disease consequences. For instance, when comparisons are made in case-control studies between persons who have a disease being investigated and persons without the disease, the control or comparison group is frequently composed of people who have another disease or who have been hospitalized. Thus when lung cancer patients are compared to other cancer patients, or patients with cancer of the cervix are compared to patients with nongenital cancers, risk factors common to both groups, such as socioeconomic status, may not emerge in analyses. In these cases the selection of the control group determines that only factors specific to one disease will appear. On the other hand, if the investigator uses healthy people as controls, a risk factor may emerge from the analyses but the investigator may not be able to determine whether it is specific to the particular disease under study or is associated with an array of conditions. Only multiple comparisons and the examining of a wide range of outcomes will help investigators assess whether a factor has specific or general disease consequences.

Another way the theory of specificity has manifested itself in medical thought is in disease classification. Diseases are generally classified first on the basis of symptomatology and ultimately on an etiologic basis. Fevers, for example, were redefined after specific causal agents were discovered. Although this certainly represents an advance from previous classification methods, factors that influence many diseases—for example, malnutrition or diseases that are multifactorial (i.e., coronary heart disease) —are troublesome, if not impossible to classify by this approach. Ultimately we need a classification system and a model of causation that can include some variables that are specific to a particular condition and others that are linked to a set of conditions. A model of disease causation should also be able to define a condition that has many causal factors interacting with one another in various ways (Cassel, 1976; Koopman, 1977; Rothman, 1976). This need is especially evident when examining diseases that are common today.

The changing health picture

Life expectancy at birth in the United States jumped from 47 years in 1900 to 68 years in 1950 (U.S., D.H.H.S., 1980). That increase in longevity, 45 percent in a half-century, reflected one of the most spectacular health advances in the history of humanity. However, it resulted almost entirely from progress against infant mortality and the communicable diseases that affect mainly young people.

From 1900 to 1960, life expectancy at age 65 increased only 2 years, from 12 to 14 years. The failure to extend life very much in the adult and later years during the first half of the century resulted mainly from the increasing occurrence of fatal chronic diseases, particularly coronary heart disease.

During the first decade or two of the second half of the twentieth century, however, health advances in early life slowed. Infant mortality, which had been dropping steadily for several decades, remained almost the same from 1955 to 1965. Meanwhile, the toll from coronary heart disease, lung cancer, and chronic respiratory disease continued to rise. During that same period the health records of several other nations, especially those of northern and western Europe, advanced substantially beyond that of the United States. Infant mortality and mortality of middle-aged men in the Scandinavian countries, for example, dropped considerably below that of the United States.

Beginning about 1965, the picture began to change again. Infant mortality resumed its decline, dropping from 25 per 1000 live births in 1965 to 13 in 1980. Coronary heart disease, first described in the United States in 1912 and rising in incidence to cause about one-third of all deaths during 1960–1965, turned sharply downward. An approximate 30 percent decline in mortality from coronary heart disease in the period 1965–1979 typified the general and substantial improvement in the U.S. mortality picture as a whole. Except for lung cancer among middle-aged and older people and violence among young people, the trend was largely favorable.

Of considerable interest was the extension of life expectancy in the later years, not just in infancy and childhood. As just noted, from 1900 to 1960 the increase at age 65 went only from 12 to 14 years. During the period 1960–1977, however, while life expectancy at birth was rising from 70 to 73 years, beginning at age 65 it increased from 14 to 16 years.

These changes in death rates and longevity stimulated reconsideration of some long-held notions about health: that the major fatal diseases of middle and later life in the second half of the twentieth century were "degenerative"; that they reflected "poor natural endowment"; and that "three-score and ten" constituted the natural limit to life for most individuals. By 1980 it seemed reasonable to expect that women would soon achieve a life expectancy at birth of 80 years, and that men might do the same in the not too distant future.

Whereas during the early 1960s it appeared that northern and western European countries were generally surpassing the health attainments of the United States, the end of the 1970s showed a different trend. The United States was rapidly overcoming the differences and in some respects the comparison countries were slipping a bit.

Infectious diseases such as influenza and pneumonia, tuberculosis, and gastroenteritis, major causes of death in 1900, account for only a small percentage of deaths in the 1980s. They have been replaced by diseases such as coronary heart disease, cancer, stroke, diabetes, and rheumatoid arthritis. Mortality among young adults is now most likely to be the result of motor vehicle accidents, violence, or suicide (Erhardt and Berlin, 1974).

These diseases are substantially different from the major diseases of earlier times, one of the most obvious differences being that they are mainly noncommunicable. They are also commonly defined as chronic illnesses because they develop very slowly, usually with advancing age. They often involve progressive damage and structural disorganization in affected organs or the entire body, causing increasing physical disability that is not easily reversible. Although some infectious diseases are chronic in nature (e.g., tuberculosis), and perhaps some additional chronic illnesses will prove to be infectious, infectious diseases tend to manifest themselves as acute episodes of illness. Furthermore, though the etiology of the noncommunicable chronic diseases is far from well understood, it is likely that many factors interact to cause them. Few "necessary" factors have yet been established.

Development of chronic disease surveys

As the nature of the diseases affecting modern populations has changed, so have the ways of measuring and defining physical health status. In the nineteenth and early twentieth centuries, the degree to which people had achieved freedom from early mortality and the major fatal diseases of the time constituted their health status. Systems for measuring the nature and extent of those problems, as well as progress against them, included death registration statistics and the compilation of data concerning reportable diseases such as cholera, typhoid fever, and tuberculosis (Lilienfeld, 1980). Infant mortality and the incidence of tuberculosis were commonly used indices of health. Trends in such conditions and their distribution among various segments of the population pinpointed the health problems and guided efforts to deal with them.

Whereas health had thus previously been defined appropriately in the negative—as the absence of disease—it appeared in the second half of the twentieth century that health was something more complex, not so easily measured as the absence of specific diseases, particularly infectious ones. Even assessing the presence or absence of chronic diseases is typically a difficult problem at the onset of the condition. Diagnosis is commonly based on somewhat arbitrary quantitative rather than qualitative changes, and it frequently entails a subjective assessment of dysfunction, disability, or discomfort. One could argue that the severity of chronic illness, especially among middle-aged and elderly people, is at least as important as its presence or absence.

Although it is clear that major changes in health status have occurred over the last 150 years, Comstock (1974) noted:

It is now difficult to realize how little was known about the health of the nation or about the health of any of its political subdivisions as recently as 50 years ago. At that time, there were only four general sources of information: death statistics, reports of notifiable diseases, prevalence of illness from two U.S. Censuses, and a few scattered surveys of illness prevalence and incidence. Each of these sources provided data that was unsatisfactory on several counts (p. 162).

For most chronic conditions, reporting procedures similar to communicable disease notification were not feasible. That fact necessitated the development of new epidemiologic methods tailored to measure the distribution, incidence, and prevalence of chronic conditions, as well as the disability and mortality associated with them. Mortality data provided an incomplete picture of the consequences of chronic disease because many conditions were not immediately, if ever, fatal. On the other hand they often involved long periods of disability and discomfort. It thus became important to develop epidemiologic methods whereby, as Sydenstricker noted in 1931, "human populations could be observed for as complete an incidence as possible of various diseases, so far as they were manifested in illness, under actual conditions of community life" (Sydenstricker, 1974). These methods of measuring morbidity in a community would chart both chronic and infectious diseases.

As a response to this problem, Frost (1941), Goldberger and colleagues (1920), and Sydenstricker (1925) began to develop new epidemiologic methods and ways to measure morbidity. Their aim was to go beyond death and particular diseases as health indices. Just as the latter indices had focused on the major health tasks of earlier days, the new efforts to measure health focused on the emerging problems of the twentieth century. Because there were greater numbers of middle-aged and older people, these problems reflected the illnesses of the older population and the factors that influenced them. The main tasks were to develop health indices that would be sensitive to chronic diseases and impairments, and also to measure disability. In addition to objective reports of severe illness or death, days lost from work, the extent of hospital or other care used, and subjective reports of health were included in the new indices of health status. The new measures of physical health included items concerning not only specific diseases but also very general conditions and infectious as well as noninfectious conditions.

Furthermore, by the mid-twentieth century it began to make sense to start thinking of health in a truly positive way, because better living conditions, greater longevity, and a higher overall level of health status were being attained in large areas of the industrialized world. Recognizing this new situation, the World Health Organization defined health as "physical, mental, and social well-being, not merely the absence of disease or infirmity" (World Health Organization, 1948). Although this definition is often criticized as being too global, difficult to use quantitatively, and idealistic, it does reflect the striving for a positive view of health. It represents a more general, non-disease-specific view of health than had been used previously.

The epidemiologic methods developed by Goldberger and Sydenstricker to measure chronic morbidity and acute illness episodes evolved in general from methods based on the study of infectious diseases. It is important to note that chronic and infectious disease are not necessarily distinct or mutually exclusive conditions. In fact, some of the "chronic" diseases first examined by these men were infectious—for example, tuberculosis—or suspected of being infectious—for example, pellagra. Perhaps the most important epidemiologic principle held in common by both infectious disease investigators and those with a growing interest in chronic conditions was to focus on geographically defined populations. Most epidemiologists, whether studying acute or chronic disease, morbidity, or mortality, sought to examine entire communities. Work on infectious diseases involved the collection of morbidity and mortality data by the reporting of these events by physicians to central agencies. Less common but still used was the household survey in which physicians or interviewers visited households and examined household members for specific diseases or asked them about disease occurrence. Both these methods allowed the epidemiologist to develop rates of disease occurrence and risks of disease, so as to compare one group to another. These methods served as the basis for studies of chronic disease morbidity.

In some ways, however, the evolving techniques and methods for measuring chronic morbid conditions were different from those used in previous epidemiologic studies. Advances in sampling techniques permitted reliable estimates of the extent and distribution of illness in a population based on information from a sample of that population. This meant that the burden of 100 percent reporting could be avoided.

Furthermore, previous studies of mortality and morbidity from infectious diseases were based largely on physicians' determinations. Physicians, or in some cases physician substitutes, certified deaths and diseases. The individual's role in the measurement process was simply to come into the hands of the physician, who made the observations and judgments and then reported them.

The physician's view of illness, however, gave only an indirect indication of a significant dimension of the health problem: disability. Only the individual affected can feel how sharp a backache is or how extensive joint stiffness is, although there may be objective evidence of disease as well as subjective reports of pain, discomfort, or disability. Putting aside exclusive reliance on physicians' judgments, investigators using morbidity survey methods adopted the view that people were ill when they said they were ill. The social impact of illness on work or other activities of ill persons is reflected in their self-perceptions and reports. These were regarded as separable from, though often closely related to, the medical classification of the phenomena. Some surveys of chronic disease and disability examined in great detail the relationships among self-reported morbidity and disability, physicians' diagnoses, and mortality in an attempt to understand the differences in health status when measured in the three different ways (Commission on Chronic Illness, 1957, 1959).

In addition to assessing the health status of communities and subgroups within communities in a descriptive way, investigators conducting the surveys frequently sought to understand the etiology of chronic diseases. Clinical impressions and mounting evidence from other sources indicated that certain behaviors and environmental conditions might have an important role in causing many chronic diseases. Thus community illness surveys often focused on social, economic, behavioral, and environmental factors and their associations with the incidence and prevalence of chronic conditions (Frost, 1941; Kasius, 1974; Terris, 1964). Prospective community studies lend themselves quite easily to assessing these types of factors, whereas other study designs such as case-control, retrospective cohort, and twin studies may be more efficient in studying some specific diseases or certain exposures and constitutional or genetic factors. There are several reasons for this:

1. In self-report surveys, respondents have the opportunity to answer questions about their behaviors and socioenvironmental conditions that may be unknown to any other sources.
2. Community studies include respondents living in many different circumstances, whereas other study designs may have built-in selection biases that exclude precisely those people one might wish to study— that is, those who are very ill at home, poor, or do not come to medical attention.
3. If the survey is done prospectively, information on important items may be obtained before the onset of illness.

Several community surveys in the United States and elsewhere were guided by this new perspective, identifying morbid conditions with socioenvironmental and behavioral characteristics as reported by people themselves. The first of these large-scale illness surveys focused extensively on a specific disease, pellagra, and its relation to dietary, social, and economic conditions. In 1916, pellagra was the second most common cause of death in South Carolina and a disease of major consequence in the southern United States. The Public Health Service sent Goldberger to investigate the disease. Through an ingenious series of studies, he identified a dietary factor, later shown to be a vitamin deficiency, as the cause of the disease (Terris, 1964). Sydenstricker and Goldberger then conducted a survey of 747 households in seven cotton-mill villages to assess the relationships among disabling illness, pellagra, diet, and economic conditions (Goldberger, et al., 1920; Sydenstricker et al., 1974). They described the impoverished conditions associated with pellagra and disabling illness, as well as the relationship between food supply and the social and economic conditions tied to the tenant farming system and single-crop agricultural production. Though Goldberger and Sydenstricker correctly identified the cause of pellagra, it was not until several decades later (during World War II) that it disappeared as an endemic disease, after socioeconomic conditions had changed and federal programs began to provide Americans with a better diet.

The surveys of cotton-mill villages, mainly short-term cross-sectional studies of a unique population, encouraged Sydenstricker to study morbidity rates in several industries (Sydenstricker and Brundage, 1974). Subsequently he decided that it was important to obtain information about all people in a community, not only those who work. He undertook the first substantial effort to measure health by means of a morbidity survey of a general population. Sydenstricker noted that this study was aimed at "recording illnesses, as ordinarily understood, that were experienced by a population group composed of persons of all ages and both sexes, and in no remarkable way unusual" (Sydenstricker, 1925).

This survey, undertaken in Hagerstown, Maryland in 1921–1924 by the U.S. Public Health Service in cooperation with the Hagerstown Health Department, included observations on 1815 households of white families. Morbidity information was collected concerning 8587 persons. Household informants interviewed every 6–8 weeks for 28 months reported both disabling and nondisabling acute and chronic illnesses for all family members. In addition, medical records were routinely collected to corroborate information given in the survey. Although the specific findings of this study are too detailed to report here, several comments are in order. One of the most striking findings was that the major causes of illness were quite different from the leading causes of death. For example, 61 percent of illnesses were due to respiratory diseases, but only 20 percent of the deaths in Hagerstown in the same period were attributable to such causes. Thus the relationship between morbidity and mortality was not a simple one. Sydenstricker also found that the completeness of the health data from the Hagerstown survey compared favorably with disease reporting in the earlier studies of industrial workers. This indicated to him that self-reports of illness might be an accurate way to assess morbidity. Finally, Sydenstricker noted the need to supplement interview data with physical and laboratory examinations of the general population in order to obtain a clearer and more complete picture of morbid conditions.

Based largely on the studies of the cotton-mill villages, industrial workers, and the community of Hagerstown, the U.S. Public health Service, often with the participation of other agencies, launched several more morbidity surveys. Between 1928 and 1931, 9000 families in 130 localities, mostly in urban areas, were asked in interviews about their illnesses and their medical and dental care (Collins, 1944). Similar surveys were launched in Cattaraugus County, in Syracuse, New York (Collins, et al., 1955), and in the Eastern District of Baltimore (Collins, et al., 1950). These three surveys each involved periodic interviews with an adult member of each household concerning cases of illness during the interval since the previous interview, acute and chronic conditions, and level of disability. Data from these three surveys, from the survey conducted in Hagerstown, and from the sickness study of 9000 families are combined in one volume (Collins, et al., 1955).

These surveys laid the foundations for the first National Health Survey in 1935–1936. From single interviews with members of 700,000 families located in 83 cities and 23 rural areas in 19 states, the National Health Survey obtained for the country as a whole data about illness that kept an individual from his or her usual activity on the day of the survey, or for 7 days during the preceding 12 months, as well as data about chronic diseases and impairments, whether disabling or not (Perrott, et al., 1939). By the mid-1940s several other countries were starting to collect information on morbidity (Slater, 1946; Committee on the Morbidity Survey, 1955).

In 1949 in the United States, the Commission on Chronic Illness decided to undertake research aimed at defining the size and nature of the chronic illness problems. Surveys of at least two communities—one urban and one rural—were recommended to assess the magnitude of the problem. In the early 1950s the commission sponsored two surveys, one in Hunterdon County, New Jersey (Commission on Chronic Illness, 1959) and one in Baltimore, Maryland (Commission on Chronic Illness, 1957).

The Hunterdon County Survey included interviews of 4426 families and a clinical evaluation of a subsample of 1569 respondents who were said to have received medical attention during the period covered by the family interview. Physicians of respondents in the subsample were contacted and asked to verify conditions as well as to report any other conditions. Thus the Hunterdon County study permitted comparisons of physicians' reports of illness with respondents' reports.

The Baltimore study, conducted similarly to the Hunterdon study, included several additional components. The survey of 11,574 individuals in more than 3500 households was supplemented with (1) a clinical evaluation of 809 respondents, (2) a screening of just over 2000 people for a wide variety of medical conditions, and (3) a vocational rehabilitation demonstration of 36 respondents.

Experience in these studies and the usefulness of data gathered made a great contribution to the establishment, in 1956, of the U.S. National Health Survey. They also paved the way for many more community surveys of chronic illness, of which the Human Population Laboratory was to be one.

Surveys of illness in communities have constituted a major innovation in epidemiologic research over the past 60 years. Effectively utilizing modern sampling techniques and principles of biostatistics, they made possible important strides in developing new measures of health status. They offered comprehensive descriptions of illness in communities and indeed, after the National Health Survey started, they were capable of describing the state of health of the entire U.S. population. With the increasing acceptance of the survey techniques in epidemiologic research, investigators moved beyond descriptive tasks to studying the etiology of the major diseases of the second half of the twentieth century.

References

Berkson J: Smoking and cancer of the lung. *Proc. Staff Meetings Mayo Clin.* 35:367–385, 1960.

Berkson J: Mortality and marital status. *Am. J. Public Health* 52:1318–1329, 1962.

Buer MC: *Health, Wealth, and Population in the Early Days of the Industrial Revolution.* London, Routledge & Kegan Paul, 1968.

Cassel J: The contribution of the social environment to host resistance. *Am. J. Epidemiol.* 104(2):107–123, 1976.

Collins SD: *The Incidence of Illness and the Volume of Medical Services Among 9,000 Canvassed Families* (collection of 23 reprints). Washington, D.C., U.S. Government Printing Office, 1944.

Collins, SD, Trantham KS, Lehmann JL: *Sickness Experience in Selected Areas of the United States.* Public Health Monograph No. 25, DHS Publ. No. 390, Washington, D.C., U.S. Government Printing Office, 1955.

Collins, SD, Phillips FR, Oliver DS: Specific causes of illness found in monthly canvasses of families: sample of the Eastern Health District of Baltimore, 1938–43. *Public Health Rep.* 65:1235–1264, 1950.

Commission on Chronic Illness: *Chronic Illness in the United States. Vol. IV.*

Chronic Illness in a Large City: The Baltimore Study. Cambridge, Mass., Harvard University Press, 1957.

Commission on Chronic Illness: *Chronic Illness in the United States. Vol. III, Chronic Illness in a Rural Area: The Hunterdon Study.* Cambridge, Mass., Harvard University Press, 1959.

Committee on the Morbidity Survey: The Danish National Morbidity Survey of 1950. *Dan. Med. Bull.* 2:148–152, 1955.

Comstock G: Commentary in Kasius RV (ed): *The Challenge of Facts: Selected Public Health Papers of Edgar Sydenstricker.* New York, Prodist, 1974.

Dubos R: *Mirage of Health.* New York, Harper and Row, 1959.

Dubos R: *Man Adapting.* New Haven, Conn., Yale University Press, 1965.

Erhardt, LL, Berlin, JE: *Mortality and Morbidity in the United States.* Cambridge, Mass., Harvard University Press, 1974.

Evans AS: Causation and disease: the Henle-Koch postulates revisited. *Yale J. Biol. Med.* 49:175–195, 1976.

Fox JP, Hall CE, Elveback LE: *Epidemiology: Man and Disease.* London, Macmillan, 1972.

Frost WH: How much control of tuberculosis? *Am. J. Public Health* 27:759–766, 1937.

Frost WH: in Maxcy KF (ed): *Papers of Wade Hampton Frost.* New York, Commonwealth Fund, 1941.

Gajdusek DC: Kuru and Creutzfeldt-Jakob disease. *Ann. Clin. Res.* 4:254–261, 1973.

Goldberger J, Wheeler GA, Sydenstricker E: A study of the relation of family income and other economic factors to pellagra incidence in seven cotton-mill villages of South Carolina in 1916. *Public Health Rep.* 35(46): 2673–2714, 1920.

Hemminki E, Paakkulainen A: The effects of antibiotics on mortality from infectious diseases in Sweden and Finland. *Am. J. Public Health* 66: 1180–1184, 1976.

Henle J: *On Miasmata and Contagie.* G Rosen (trans), Baltimore, Johns Hopkins Press, 1933.

Henle J, Henle W, Diehl V: Relation of Burkitts tumor-associated herpes-types virus to infectious mononucleosis. *Proc. Ntl. Acad. Sci. USA* 59:94–100, 1968.

Hippocrates: *The Genuine Works of Hippocrates.* F Adams (trans), Baltimore, Williams & Wilkins, 1938, pp. 19–41.

Kasius RV (ed): *The Challenge of Facts: Selected Public Health Papers of Edgar Sydenstricker.* New York, Prodist, 1974.

Koch R: Verber bakteriologische Forschung. *Verhandlungen des X. Internationalen Medizinischen Kongresses Berlin,* 4–9 August 1890, 35–47 Berlin, Hirschwald.

Koopman JS: Causal models and sources of interaction. *Am. J. Epidemiol.* 106(6): 439–444, 1977.

Krause AK: Tuberculosis and public health. *Am. Rev. Tuberculosis* 18:271–322, 1928.

Lilienfeld AM: *Foundations of Epidemiology.* New York, Oxford University Press, 1980.

Linenthal H: Sanitation of clothing factories and tenement-house work-rooms, in Locke EA (ed): *Tuberculosis in Massachusetts,* Boston, Wright & Potter, 1908, pp. 28–36.

Mausner JS, Bahn AK: *Epidemiology: An Introductory Text.* Philadelphia, W. B. Saunders Co., 1974.

McKeown T: A historical appraisal of the medical task, in McLachlan G, McKeown T (eds): *Medical History and Medical Care.* London, Oxford University Press for the Nuffield Provincial Hospitals Trust, 1971.

McKeown T: *The Role of Medicine: Dream, Mirage, or Nemesis?* London, Nuffield Provincial Hospitals Trust, 1976.

Newberne PM, Williams G: Nutritional influence on the course of infections, in Dunlop RH, Moon HW (eds): *Resistance to Infectious Disease.* Saskatoon, Sask., Saskatoon Modern Press, 1970.

Park WH, Schroeder MC, Zingher A: The control of diphtheria. *Am. J. Public Health* 13:23–32, 1923.

Perrott G, Tibbits C, Britten RH: The national health survey—scope and method of nationwide canvass of sickness in relation to its social and economic setting. *Public Health Rep.* 54:1663–1687, 1939.

Porter RR: The contribution of the biological and medical sciences to human welfare, presented at Swansea Meeting, The British Association for the Advancement of Science, 1972, pp. 95–101.

Powles J: On the limitations of modern medicine. *Science, Medicine and Man* 1:1–30, 1973.

Rosen G: *Preventive Medicine in the United States: 1900–1975.* New York, Science History Publications, 1975.

Rothman KV: Causes. *Am. J. Epidemiol.* 104:587–592, 1976.

Semmelweis IP: The etiology, the concept, and the prophylaxis of childbed fever. FB Murphy (trans), *Medical Classics* 5:350–733, 1941.

Sigerist H: *The Great Doctors.* New York, W.W. Norton, 1933.

Slater P: *Survey of Sickness, October 1943 to December 1945. The Social Survey.* London, Her Majesty's Stationery Office, 1946.

Snow J: On the mode of communication of cholera, in Snow J (ed): *Snow on Cholrea.* New York: Commonwealth Fund 1936, pp. 1–175.

Stewart GT: Limitations of the germ theory. *Lancet* 1:1077–1081, 1968.

Susser M: *Causal Thinking in the Health Sciences: Concepts and Strategies in Epidemiology.* New York, Oxford University Press, 1973.

Susser M: Judgment and causal inference: criteria in epidemiologic studies. *Am. J. Epidemiol.* 105(1):1–15, 1977.

Sydenstricker E: The incidence of illness in a general population group. General results of a morbidity study from December 1, 1921 through March 31, 1924, in Hagerstown, Md. *Public Health Rep.* 40:279–291, 1925.

Sydenstricker E: Statistics of morbidity, in Kasius RV (ed): *The Challenge of Facts: Selected Public Health Papers of Edgar Sydenstricker.* New York, Prodist, 1974, pp. 228–245.

Sydenstricker E, Brundage DK: Industrial establishment disability records as a source of morbidity statistics, in Kasius RV (ed): *The Challenge of Facts: Selected Public Health Papers of Edgar Sydenstricker.* New York, Prodist, 1974, pp. 186–203.

Sydenstricker E, Wheeler A, Goldberger J: Disabling sickness among the population of seven cotton-mill villages of South Carolina in relation to family income, in Kasius RV (ed): *The Challenge of Facts: Selected Public Health Papers of Edgar Sydenstricker*. New York, Prodist, 1974, pp. 168–185.

Syme SL, Berkman LF: Social class, susceptibility, and sickness. *Am. J. Epidemiol.* **104**(1):1–8, 1976.

Terris M: *Goldberger on Pellagra*. Baton Rouge, La., Louisiana State University Press, 1964.

United States, Dept. of Health and Human Services: *Health in the United States*. Publ. No. (PHS) 81-1232, 1980.

World Health Organization: Test of the constitution of World Health Organization. *Official Records WHO* **2**:100, 1948.

Yerushalmy J, Palmer CE: On the methodology of investigations of etiologic factors in chronic diseases. *J. Chron. Dis.* **10**:27–40, 1959.

Zingher A: Diphtheria preventive work in public schools of New York City. *Arch. Pediatrics* **38**:336–359, 1921.

2. The human population laboratory: history, concepts, methods

Inspired in large part by the community surveys of morbidity, the California State Department of Public Health started a chronic disease program in the late 1940s. That required estimating the nature and extent of chronic conditions in California.

As a first step in this direction, the department established a Tumor Registry in 1947 in order to guide public health efforts to deal with that important chronic disease. The California Tumor Registry was based on reporting and follow-up of cancer cases seen in selected hospitals in 1942 and thereafter. In 1960 it was extended to cover all of Alameda County, and in 1970 to the entire San Francisco Bay area. The Tumor Registry was and continues to be useful in many respects, such as in evaluating the effectiveness of treatment modalities for various forms of cancer. That pattern, however, proved inapplicable to the chronic disease problem as a whole. One difficulty is that a registry does not provide a base for studying prospectively the development of chronic illness and of factors contributing to disease incidence, although it can serve as a resource for ascertaining outcomes in such studies. A second problem is that many cases of chronic disease are difficult to diagnose and do not consistently come to hospitals or, in fact, any medical attention. Finally, though it might be possible to establish similar registries for a few more chronic diseases, covering all such diseases in that fashion would obviously be too burdensome.

With support from the federal government, the State Department of

Public Health initiated a Morbidity Research Project in 1949. The aim was to develop a measure of morbidity in the general population that would be useful both in establishing services to deal with chronic diseases and in guiding further studies. A pilot morbidity survey in San Jose, California, was the initial step. The chief aims of that venture were to test the feasibility of methods for collecting morbidity information and to assess the reliability and validity of the methods. Successful completion of that pilot study led to the decision to embark upon a statewide survey in California during 1954–1955, using the sample household interview method. That California study and similar studies conducted elsewhere laid the groundwork for the National Health Survey mentioned in Chapter 1.

Purpose of the human population laboratory

With the completion of these preliminary surveys investigators in the Bureau of Chronic Diseases, California State Department of Public Health, began to focus on two broad issues. The first was how to conceptualize and measure health status in a way that would be consistent with the World Health Organization (WHO) definition of health: "physical, mental and social well-being, not merely the absence of disease and infirmity." Many thought this definition was too vague to be useful for scientific purposes. The group sought to measure health along a spectrum from negative to positive, that is, from death, disability, and illness to positive well-being.

The second issue the investigators wanted to study was how certain ways of living (including personal habits as well as familial, cultural, economic, social, and environmental factors) affected health. Although many of these ways of living had not been strongly linked to physical health by previous studies, indications were growing that they might play an important role in determining health status in modern industrialized countries.

The National Institutes of Health in 1959, with the endorsement of peer-review bodies, allocated funds to establish a Human Population Laboratory (HPL) in Berkeley with three long-term objectives:

1. To assess the level of health (including physical, mental, and social dimensions) of persons living in Alameda County, California
2. To ascertain whether particular levels in one dimension of health tend to be associated with comparable levels in other dimensions
3. To determine relationships of various ways of living and selected demographic characteristics to levels of health

The third objective, that is, to study the influence of certain ways of living—specifically, common health practices and social relationships—on physical health status, constitutes the focus of this monograph.

A planning grant from the National Institutes of Health permitted recruitment of a multidisciplinary group from epidemiology, sociology, psychology, statistics, and other fields pertinent to the project. Work has continued steadily for 20 years, with three of the main investigators involved throughout that period of time.

Concept and methods development

During the early years of the Human Population Laboratory, concepts and methods had to be formulated and tested. This required communication among staff with quite varied backgrounds, reconciliation of differing viewpoints and implementation of agreements reached, within the limits of practicality and cost. Debate was lively. As fieldwork got under way, the group became more of a team.

The first problem encountered by the Human Population Laboratory staff was to grasp the WHO definition and convert it into operational terms for the purposes of measurement. According to this definition, the staff proposed that at any given time every person falls at some point on each of the three dimensions of health: physical, mental, and social. That series of points was to be ascertained for all persons representing a general population, in this case a sample of adults from Alameda County. This county was selected for the study because (1) its population was reasonably typical, though not statistically representative, of people in the state and nation; and (2) several health study resources, such as a Tumor Registry and medical records, including those of a large prepayment health plan, were available in the county. Also, the physical base from which the work would be conducted, the Berkeley office of the California State Department of Public Health, was located in the county.

Human Population Laboratory investigators developed separate approaches to the measurement of physical, mental, and social well-being with a view toward ultimately combining them in some fashion.

While these conceptual matters were being thrashed out, work on methods for the project started. How would individuals be selected to represent the adult population of Alameda County? How were the data to be collected in order to place each individual on three spectra of health, and to reveal determinants of that placement? What could be done to enhance reliability and validity of the data?

The group decided that an area probability sample would be the most feasible way of representing the area's adult population, provided a satisfactory rate of response could be obtained. Individuals were to be selected through a household-sampling frame to represent all noninstitutionalized persons over 20 years of age living in the county. A questionnaire was to be designed and administered in the most economical manner consistent with the collection of good-quality data, giving particular attention to reliability and validity. A description of the sampling process and other methods appears in the following sections.

Before embarking on the extensive data-gathering process, the Human Population Laboratory carried out a series of preliminary studies in order to arrive at the best data-collection method. One question was: How could health best be assessed for purposes of the study—by having physicians examine people, or by asking people directly about their health? Though the former would be preferable for ascertaining the presence of particular diseases and certain other aspects of health, directly asking people about the conditions that constituted their physical, mental, and social health seemed the preferable way of assessing health status for this study. That determination was based not only on logistical considerations but also on conceptual grounds, namely, that systematically querying all persons in the sample would provide the best information for placing them on an illness–health spectrum.

For the exploratory field studies, approximately 2000 households in Alameda County, 1 per 150 residences, were chosen and their occupants enumerated in 1961. The first methodologic studies, in 1962, demonstrated a good response rate. Enumeration—that is, the compilation of basic demographic data on each household member—was completed in 97 percent of the occupied households. Ninety percent of the enumerated sample then responded to the health questionnaire. The early field studies focused on comparing three different strategies of data collection with respect to relative rate of return, completeness of return, cost, and validity of data.

Of the three traditional methods of collecting information from individuals—namely, personal interview, telephone interview, and self-administered mail questionnaire—the personal interview was generally believed at the time to have the highest response rate, although it was the most expensive. Telephone interviews were less expensive but were known to suffer from sampling inadequacies, whereas the least expensive mail questionnaires were said to be handicapped by relatively low response rates.

The Human Population Laboratory investigated the possibility of combining the best features of the three strategies of data collection by actually testing them in the field. The "personal interview strategy" started with personal contacts, with telephone and mail follow-up as needed; in the "telephone strategy" the initial telephone contact was supplemented with personal and mail inquiries; and in the "mail strategy," mail questionnaires were followed by telephone and personal interviews.

All three strategies yielded highly comparable response rates. Furthermore, the proportion of questions left unanswered was about the same, only 2 percent higher in the mail than in the other strategies. Most important, the findings from the three strategies were virtually interchangeable. Thus the quality of the data was about the same. The major difference was in cost per completed questionnaire: the personal interview strategy was more than twice as expensive as the mail strategy (Hochstim, 1962, 1967, 1970). These results and findings from other exploratory studies gave the investigators sufficient confidence in the "mail strategy" to adopt it as the basic data-collection method for the larger survey.

The Human Population Laboratory staff also conducted an investigation of cervical cytology in 1962, with a view to testing the methodology on a current health problem. There was a 91 percent response rate, and 87 percent agreement between the respondent and the medical sources named as to whether a Papanicolaou smear had been performed. The findings indicated that information significant to health could be collected by mail questionnaire and that the data could be of value in guiding services: an important preventive medical service was then being used by a substantial portion of the population, mostly by the relatively affluent, who suffered less from the disease. The poor who needed it most used the cytology service the least (Breslow and Hochstim, 1964).

Data from the 1962 survey also permitted examination of the interrelationships of race, income, and geographic (poverty) area of residence to health and health care. People with higher incomes living in non-poverty areas were found to enjoy better health and health care than those with lower incomes. Even at the same income level, however, poverty area residents had more health problems than those outside poverty areas (Hochstim et al., 1968).

Because the Human Population Laboratory was to be a prospective study in which the respondents were to be followed through subsequent interviews as well as through mortality checks, it was important to ascertain the extent to which one could expect to make contact with persons surveyed after a lapse of some years. A follow-up in 1964 of the population enumerated in 1961 disclosed that 40 percent of the persons had changed their residence within the past 3 years. Two-thirds of those who moved, however, were still in Alameda County, and three-fourths within the San Francisco Bay metropolitan area. A relocation effort reached 91 percent of the nonrespondents not known to have died.

After these pilot surveys in the early 1960s, the first definitive survey questionnaire went to a larger random sample of men and women in Alameda County in 1965.

In 1974, a follow-up survey was conducted among the 1965 respondents; also, a new random sample of adults in the community in 1974 provided a cross-sectional view as of that time. Mortality data were collected for the 9-year period between the 1965 and 1974 surveys. Thus analysis of the items from the 1965 and 1974 surveys yields cross-sectional information on the health status of that adult population of the county at those times, and on factors possibly related to health status. The 1965 survey, coupled with the 9-year mortality follow-up of that sample, provides prospective informa-tion on the relationship of various social, psychological, and environ-mental factors to mortality. Analyses of the responses to the two surveys also permit longitudinal study of a wide variety of issues, such as the effects of social and behavioral factors on changes in physical health status. Finally, comparisons of community responses to the 1965 and 1974 surveys cast light on changes in health, demographic, and other char-acteristics that occurred in the community between the two survey periods.

Profile of Alameda County:
The community setting

Alameda County, part of the San Francisco-Oakland standard metro-politan area, included in 1965 a population of approximately one million, almost entirely urban or suburban. Between 1940 and 1965, Alameda County's population had almost doubled; most of this growth took place in the southern part of the county (California State Dept. of Health, 1966). In 1940, only 21 percent of the population lived in the South county. By 1965, however, the South county included 49 percent of the population and by 1970, 54 percent. This increase was typical of many areas of the country in which the size of populations in the central cities remained relatively stable while suburban and urban fringe areas showed major population gains. Figures 2-1 and 2-2 illustrate these trends.

Among Alameda County residents in 1965, 82 percent were white; 14 percent were black, clustered largely in the older urban centers of the North; and 4 percent were members of other races. The largest city, Oakland, was 30 percent black, and Berkeley–Albany 21 percent black; South county, on the other hand, was almost entirely white. Alameda County's black population was growing somewhat faster than that of California as a whole. The sharpest increase occurred during World War II, when blacks came to the East Bay counties to work in defense industries, but in-migration continued thereafter.

Between 1940 and 1965 the age distribution of Alameda County's population shifted toward the young, with the proportion of persons under 20 years of age growing from 26 percent to 38 percent. As elsewhere

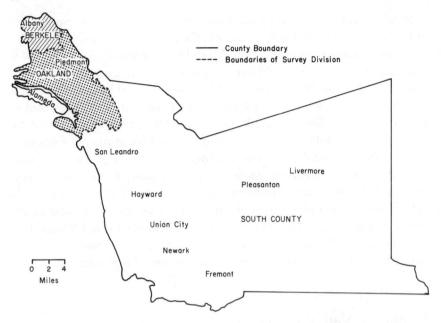

Fig. 2-1. Major subdivisions of Alameda County. (*From* California State Dept. of Public Health: *Alameda County Population 1965*; 1966.)

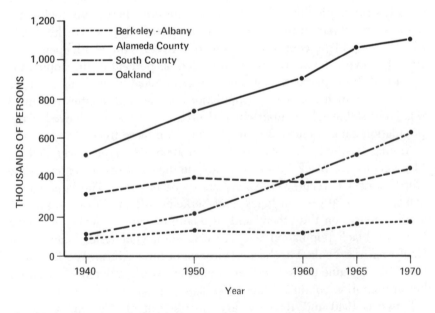

Fig. 2-2. Population trends for Alameda County and major subdivisions, 1940–1970.

in the country, suburbanites in Alameda County were generally younger than residents of the central cities, Oakland and Berkeley–Albany.

Among the population 20 and over, 68 percent were married, 18 percent single, and the remaining 14 percent widowed, separated, or divorced. Women were more likely than men to be widowed, separated, or divorced —especially older women. Also, blacks were more likely than whites to be separated or divorced.

Alameda County's mid-1965 unemployment rate was 3.9 percent of the male civilian labor force and 5.5 percent of the female labor force. At that same time the national unemployment rate was 4.1 percent for males and 5.6 percent for females. The population groups most heavily affected by unemployment in Alameda County, as elsewhere, were the young (16–24), blacks, unskilled workers, single people (most of whom are young), and separated or divorced persons. Of the male working population, 15 percent were in professional occupations, 12 percent were in managerial positions, 17 percent were in clerical and sales work, 22 percent were craftsmen or foremen, 18 percent were operatives, and 16 percent were either service workers or laborers.

Demographic differences between Oakland and the southern part of Alameda County were similar to those noted in other American cities and their surrounding suburban and rural areas. Oakland had a higher percentage of elderly white people, a building vacancy rate twice as high, twice the rate of separated and divorced people, and over three times the proportion of children living in one-parent families. Such statistics resulted in several parts of the city being designated as "target areas" for federal antipoverty programs (Hochstim, et al., 1968).

Thus Alameda County is not a homogeneous community. It includes growing suburbs and troubled inner-city areas; people in various economic and occupational strata; young and old; married and single; and people of several racial and ethnic groups. Though not representative of all America, Alameda County is typical of the largely industrialized, urbanized areas of the country.

Sample design and data collection in 1965

Data for the Human Population Laboratory come from people selected to represent the adult population of Alameda County, based on a two-stage stratified systematic sample of Alameda County housing units. The sample excluded persons living in hospitals, prisons, and other institutions, as well as persons living in Alameda County only temporarily with a permanent address elsewhere. Within groups of three housing units, demographic information such as age, race, sex, and employment status was gathered for all occupants.

Taking costs and precision into account, investigators prepared the survey sample to include 4000 to 5000 households. Selection of a 4000-household sample on the basis of the 1960 county population would produce the sampling fraction:

$$\frac{n}{N} = \frac{4000}{310,312} = \frac{1}{77.6}$$

This sampling fraction applied to the 1965 population was expected to yield somewhat more than 4000 households.

Sampling required three steps:

1. Stratification of Alameda County
2. Selection of blocks from each stratum
3. Selection of housing units within each block

Based on 1960 Census data, Alameda County was stratified into 25 categories. These contained approximately equal numbers of housing units and were composed of contiguous census tracts that varied in geographic size. The strata were designed to maximize homogeneity within strata and differences between strata, according to median household income of census tracts.

From a listing of housing units in every block from the 1960 Census, 40 blocks were selected from each stratum. This procedure produced a total of 1000 blocks from the 25 strata. Census block statistics were available for 85 percent of all housing units in Alameda County. Selection of the remaining 15 percent of the housing units was based on Census Enumeration Districts, the smallest areas for which statistics were reported. Human Population Laboratory staff members cruised the sample enumeration districts, counted the number of housing units in these blocks, and prepared a listing from which blocks were chosen with a probability of selection proportionate to their size. Thus larger blocks had a greater chance of being selected.

Housing units were selected from sample blocks to reflect changes in population between 1960, when units were last identified in the census, and 1965 when the survey was conducted. The net result of the sampling procedure was a listing of 4735 households. As shown in Table 2-1, 283 of the total 4735 households were vacant. Among the 4452 occupied eligible housing units, enumeration was completed for 4337, or approximately 97 percent.

Within each household all persons over 20 years of age or ever married were counted in the sample, yielding a total of 8083 adult persons.

Based on the strategy developed in the preliminary field studies, respondents were asked to fill out a questionnaire and return it by mail. The

Table 2-1. Rate of return of household enumeration

Sample status	Housing units	
	No.	Percentage
Sample status of addresses		
Total number of addresses listed	4735	100.0
Vacancies	283	6.0
Occupied eligible housing units	4452	94.0
Sample status of housing units		
Total occupied eligible housing units	4452	100.0
Enumeration completed	4337	97.4
Enumeration not completed because of		
Objective refusal (ill, senile, religious reason)	12	0.3
Subjective refusal (lack of time, distrust, "invasion of privacy")	81	1.8
Not at home after repeated calls	22	0.5

From California State Dept. of Public Health: *Alameda County Population 1965*, April 1966, p. 79.

enumerator left for each adult household member a questionnaire accompanied by an explanatory letter and a stamped, self-addressed envelope, with a request that it be filled in and mailed as soon as possible, but in any case within the week. Two further attempts (one by letter and a second one either by certified letter or telegram) were made to obtain responses by mail. After this, interviewers were sent to the homes of nonrespondents to retrieve completed questionnaires or to help in their completion. Using this mail strategy (see Table 2-2), questionnaires were secured from 6928 persons, or 86 percent of the 8083 listed adults.

Accurate assessment of the bias resulting from nonresponse of some members of the sample is usually difficult, if not impossible, in such

Table 2-2. Rates of questionnaire return at successive stages of follow-up

Sample status of individuals	Adults	
	No.	Percentage
Total adults in occupied eligible housing units	8083	100.0
Returned questionnaire		
After enumeration	3358	42.0
After letter	1396	17.0
After telegram	876	11.0
After personal interview	1298	16.0
Total questionnaires returned	6928	86.0
Total questionnaires not returned	1155	14.0

surveys. In this case, however, previous enumeration of everyone in the sample makes it possible to describe the nonrespondents, compare them with respondents, and calculate the bias at least for certain demographic and socioeconomic characteristics (Hochstim, 1970). As seen in Table 2-3, the nonrespondents were older, and accordingly they were somewhat more likely to be retired and widowed. Nonrespondents were also more likely than respondents to be white and male. Nonrespondents, however, constituted only 14 percent of the enumeration sample, and their omission had very little effect on the sample estimates for the 13 characteristics for which enumeration data are available (Hochstim, 1970).

Thus, so far as it could be measured, nonresponse bias was slight. It can reasonably be assumed that the questionnaire returns fairly represent the sample.

Table 2-3. Selected characteristics of total enumerated sample respondents and non-respondents

Selected characteristics	Total enumerated	Questionaire	Nonrespondents
Total No. of persons	8083	6928	1155
Sex			
Male	46.1%	45.6%	49.4%
Female	53.9	54.4	50.6
Age (years)			
Under 30	22.5	23.7	15.5
30–44	31.5	32.2	27.5
45–64	32.3	31.3	38.6
65 and over	13.6	12.8	18.5
Race			
White	84.4	83.6	89.1
Black	12.0	12.4	9.2
Other	3.7	4.1	1.7
Marital status			
Married	74.2	74.5	72.1
Single	10.3	10.1	11.6
Separated or divorced	8.2	8.5	6.9
Widowed	7.3	7.0	9.0
Employment status			
Employed	57.8	58.2	55.2
Looking for work	2.5	2.6	1.9
Retired	8.1	7.7	10.4
Other (students, housewives, etc.)	31.6	31.5	32.3

From Hochstim, J.R.: Health and Ways of Living: The Alameda County Population Laboratory. In Kessler, I.J., Levin, M.L. (eds.): *The Community as an Epidemiological Laboratory.* Baltimore, Johns Hopkins University Press, 1970, p. 159.

It is of interest to examine what would have happened if data collection had been cut off short of the personal-contact wave. What kinds of persons were brought into the sample through this final wave? Does their inclusion change the estimates appreciably, and if so, does it consistently improve the estimates?

Table 2-4 shows estimates based on one, two, three, and all four waves of questionnaire returns, and, for comparison, the parameters derived from the enumeration. For simplicity, Table 2-4 includes only a single category of each of the 13 characteristics. The selected category is usually the one with the largest bias, or one associated with low socioeconomic status. The second wave (reminder letter) improved virtually all of the

Table 2-4. Selected demographic characteristics at cumulative stages of response and enumeration

Selected characteristics	After enumeration	After reminder letter	After telegram	Including personal contact	Enumeration
No. of Adults	3358	4754	5630	6928	8083
Females	55.2%	54.6%	54.2%ᵃ	54.4%	53.9%
65 years of age and over	14.8	13.8	12.4	12.8	13.6
Black	8.0	9.3	10.9	12.4	12.0
Presently separated or divorced	8.2	8.0	8.3	8.5	8.2
Presently looking for work	2.0	2.4	2.4	2.6	2.5
Service workers and laborers	13.2	13.3	13.8	15.1	15.1
In household with no employed persons	18.2	16.7	15.4	15.5	15.8
In rented quarters	39.3	38.4	38.5	39.5	38.8
In one- or two-room household	4.9	4.1	3.9	4.0	3.8
In household with children	48.6	50.9	52.1	53.0	51.6
In household with five or more persons	19.2	20.6	21.4	22.3	21.8
In household with more than one person per room (crowded)	4.6	5.4	6.2	7.2	7.1
In household with no telephone	5.6	5.5	6.1	6.8	7.0

ᵃEstimates closest to enumeration are underlined.

From Hochstim, J.R. and Athanasopoulos, D.A.: Personal follow-up in a mail survey: Its contribution and its cost. *Public Opinion Quarterly* 34:69–81, 1970.

estimates. Likewise, the third wave of mail returns, those obtained in response to telegrams, improved 11 of the 13 estimates. However, the effect of the final wave of returns, which was collected by sending staff members to the respondents' homes, was not consistent.

Before the fourth stage, with only the mail returns in, the sample estimates were all within 2 percentage points of the enumeration, but the following five parameters were significantly low: the percentage of adults who were over 65, were black, were service workers or laborers, were living in households that were crowded, and had no telephone. The personal-contact wave improved all five of these estimates; the mean improvement was about 1.0 percentage point. Two variables were left essentially unchanged. However, the four-wave estimates for the six other measured variables were slightly worse than those based solely on mail returns, by about 0.6 percentage points on the average.

The personal-contact wave tended to improve estimates associated with low socioeconomic status because this stratum is relatively unlikely to respond by mail; however, it also introduced some not-at-home bias characteristic of surveys conducted by personal interview, with the result that the final sample was slightly overweighted with people in large families, and with women.

For the data not collected at the time of enumeration—that is, the substantive information on health and way of living collected in the mail questionnaire—distributions are not known because 14 percent of the enumerated sample did not respond to the questionnaire. Therefore, there is no precise way of assessing the nonresponse bias for this data.

Ordinarily one might assume that the best estimate for the substantive data is the accumulated response of all persons from whom questionnaires were obtained, including those where personal retrieval was necessary. Because personal contact did improve the estimates of race and socioeconomic status to some degree, the total questionnaire returns on the substantive variables related to race and socioeconomic status in the total return are likely closest to the truth. Most of the differences in enumeration variables, however, were relatively minor.

Table 2-5 shows the accumulated responses to selected items on various subjects covered in the questionnaire. The most striking feature of this table is the close similarity among successive stages of data collection and particularly the similarities between mail responses alone and the total response, including personal contact. Among the 40 items included, the difference between mail and total returns never reached 2 percentage points, and exceeded one percentage point in only five cases. The small magnitude of the changes brought about by the personal-contact wave is in great part a function of relative weight.

The largest difference between mail and total response occurred in two categories:

1. Group activities—people who reported no organizational membership and those who indicated no political activity were less likely than others to respond by mail.
2. Socioeconomic characteristics—people with low education, job insecurity, and without provision for medical care were less likely than others to respond by mail.

The group activity items suggested that people who do not participate in community life are relatively reluctant to respond by mail. Other items indicate that the underlying factor may be low morale, leading to isolation, nonparticipation, and withdrawal: health self-rated "fair" or "poor"; "bothered" by ailment, chronic condition, or impairment; "not too happy these days"; many more negative feelings than positive; unhappy marriage; and no friends or relatives seen regularly. Again, the differences between mail and total response are small. In several cases, however, they are statistically significant, and worth noting for the possibility that persons suffering from this sort of psychological malaise may be relatively inaccessible to surveys conducted entirely by mail.

Comparison between the questionnaire returns and total enumerated sample shows that the major improvement made by the interview wave is in race and related socioeconomic distributions. Although percentage differences are small and the directions of bias not entirely consistent, the substantive results generally show a pattern congruent with that of the enumerated data: persons who were deprived, insecure, or suffering from illness were also less likely to respond by mail. In sample survey investigations based largely on mail response, perhaps even the very small improvement made by personal contacts is worthwhile.

Questionnaire content and the development of measures of health and ways of living

As noted earlier, the Human Population Laboratory study of health and ways of living accepted as a starting point the World Health Organization definition of health: "physical, mental, and social well-being, not merely the absence of disease and infirmity" (Breslow, 1972).

Thus physical health was examined in terms of general states of being well or sick, as well as in terms of specific diseases, discomforts, or disabilities. The major indicators of physical health included in the questionnaire fell into five categories: (1) energy level, compared with peers; (2) recurrent symptoms, such as headaches, coughing, pains in the

Table 2-5. Selected characteristics at cumulative stages of response

Selected characteristics	Questionnaire only	After reminder letter	After telegram	Total questionnaire response
All adults	3358	4754	5630	6928
Health				
High blood pressure	10.7%	10.5%	10.5%	10.7%
Arthritis or rheumatism	15.0	15.1	14.7	14.6
One or more chronic conditions	37.3	37.4	37.1	36.8
Bothered by chronic conditions	7.9	7.7	7.7	8.1
One or more ailments	64.1	63.8	63.3	62.6
One or more impairments	10.1	9.7	9.3	9.2
Bothered by impairments	3.2	3.1	2.9	3.1
Some disability	15.0	15.2	14.7	14.8
Report health "fair" or "poor"	16.4	17.7	17.9	18.5
Less energy than most people their age	27.6	28.5	28.8	28.5
Cannot relax easily	19.2	18.9	19.2	19.4
Often work out at the end of day	12.3	12.7	13.3	13.1
Health care				
More than 10 doctor visits during last year	9.6	9.4	9.0	9.1
Never had a medical checkup	10.6	11.0	11.4	12.3
No regular doctor	20.9	20.9	21.1	22.1
No health insurance	14.1	14.3	14.6	15.7
No health insurance and no medical or dental checkup within last year	4.7	5.1	5.2	5.8
Socioeconomic				
Grade school or less	15.7	16.2	16.6	18.1
Income less than $4000 a year	15.4	15.3	14.8	15.2
Received one or more types of welfare benefits	8.6	8.2	8.3	8.7
Financial position worse than expected	23.5	24.1	24.6	24.5
Unemployed 7 or more months in the last 2 years	7.9	8.1	8.4	8.7
Not too good in job	20.1	21.6	22.0	22.5
Not satisfied with job	7.6	7.7	8.1	8.2
Sometimes or frequently worry about keeping job	22.6	23.4	23.6	22.4
Psychological				
Not too happy these days	10.5	10.9	10.9	11.0
High anomy score	20.6	21.4	22.2	22.8
High neurotic traits score	26.1	27.1	27.4	27.3
Low ego resiliency score	32.9	33.1	33.2	33.0
Many more negative than positive feelings	12.4	12.5	12.5	12.9
Marital				
Married two or more times	19.0	18.8	19.6	20.3
Divorced one or more times	22.5	22.2	23.1	23.7

Table 2-5. (Continued)

Selected characteristics	Questionnaire only	After reminder letter	After telegram	Total questionnaire response
Considered marriage unhappy	15.1	16.8	17.6	18.0
Seriously considered divorce or separation	6.6	6.9	7.2	7.5
Group activities				
No organizational membership	28.6	28.2	28.5	30.0
Engaged in no political activity	13.9	16.4	15.7	17.4
No friends or relatives seen regularly	8.2	8.0	7.7	8.0

From Hochstim, J.R. and Athanasopoulos, D.A.: Personal follow-up in a mail survey: Its contribution and its cost. *Public Opinion Quarterly* 34:69–81, 1970.

stomach; (3) chronic conditions, such as cancer, heart trouble, and arthritis; (4) impairments, including difficulty in seeing or hearing, or a missing limb; and (5) disability, defined as a reported restriction of movement, work capacity, or other activity. All this information was collected by self-reports on the questionnaire. No medical examinations were conducted or medical records examined for purposes of determining health status. Other responses indicating degree of physical health included whether the respondent was seriously bothered by an impairment, condition, or symptom; whether the respondent believed his or her health was good, fair, or poor; and how it compared with that perceived in others of the same age as the respondent.

Many of these items describing physical health were combined into an overall index of physical well-being based on (1) current ability to perform certain usual daily activities, (2) presence during the last 12 months of one or more listed chronic conditions or impairments, (3) presence during the last 12 months of one or more listed symptoms, and (4) subjective rating of current general energy level. These four sets of items appeared to differentiate levels of health along the spectrum of physical health. Table 2-6 outlines the categories in the physical health spectrum, and shows the specific questions and lists of conditions used to differentiate the population according to the Physical Health Index.

Because there is no absolute criterion against which the spectrum can be evaluated, the categories were established largely on a priori grounds. Persons who reported limitation in their ability to perform such basic daily activities as feeding and dressing themselves or getting outdoors, or incapacity to work, comprised the poorest-health end of the spectrum. Following are those who reported curtailing hours or type of work or recreational activities because of illness or injury. Those who did not re-

Table 2-6. Categories of a Physical Health Spectrum based on questions as to disability impairments, chronic conditions, symptoms, and energy level

Category	Questions
Disability—severe 1. Reported trouble with feeding, dressing, climbing stairs, getting outdoors, or inability to work for 6 months or longer.	"Here is a list of activities that people sometimes have trouble with: trouble feeding themselves, trouble dressing themselves, trouble moving around. Do you have trouble doing any of these things?" "Here are two more activities that people sometimes have trouble with: trouble climbing stairs and trouble getting outdoors. Do you have trouble doing either of these things?" "Are you now unable to work because of some illness or injury?"
Disability—less 2. Did not report (1) above, but reported changing hours or type of work or cutting down on other activities for 6 months or longer.	"Have you had to change the kind of work you used to do, or had to cut down on the number of hours you used to work because of some illness or injury?" "Have you had to cut down or stop any other activity you used to do because of some illness or injury?"
Chronic conditions 3. Did not report any disability, but reported two or more impairments or chronic conditions in the past 12 months. 4. Did not report any disability, but reported one chronic condition or impairment in the past 12 months.	"Here is a list of medical conditions that usually last for some time. Have you had any of these conditions during the past 12 months? High blood pressure, heart trouble, stroke, chronic bronchitis, asthma, arthritis or rheumatism, epilepsy, diabetes, cancer, tuberculosis, stomach ulcer or duodenal ulcer, chronic gallbladder trouble, chronic liver trouble, hernia, or rupture. Here is a list of physical impairments. Do you have any of these? Missing hand, arm, foot, or leg. Trouble with seeing (even with glasses). Trouble with hearing (even with hearing aid). Do you have any other medical condition, ailment, or impairment that has not been listed so far? Describe it here."
Symptomatic 5. Did not report any disability, impairment, or chronic condition, but reported one or more symptoms in the past 12 months.	"Here is a list of physical ailments. Have you had any of these during the past 12 months? Frequent cramps in the legs; pain in the heart or tightness or heaviness in the chest; trouble breathing or shortness of breath; swollen ankles; pains in the back or spine; repeated pain in the stomach; frequent headaches; constant coughing or frequent heavy chest colds; paralysis of any kind; stiffness, swelling, or aching in any joint or muscle; getting very tired in a short time?"
Without complaints 6. Low to medium energy level— fewer than three high-energy answers to these questions 7. High energy level—at least three high-energy answers	"Would you say you have more energy or less energy than most people your age?" "How often do you have any trouble getting to sleep or staying asleep?" "When you have only 4 or 5 hours of sleep during the night how tired do you feel the next day?" "How often are you completely worn out at the end of the day?"

port such limitations but who reported two or more serious chronic conditions were placed next along the spectrum, and then persons with only one.
The following category included those who reported no disability or
chronic condition but did report one or more symptoms. Finally, among
the group who reported no limitations, chronic conditions, or symptoms at
all are some whose subjective rating of high energy level placed them in
the most healthy category.

There have been many problems with the criticisms of general health
status indices (Balinsky and Berger, 1975; Elinson, 1976; Goldsmith, 1972),
and the Human Population Laboratory index is not exempt from them.
The most troublesome problem is that, at this stage of conceptual development, value judgments must enter into the creation of indices
(Goldsmith, 1972). Considerable disagreement exists concerning the judgments.

In the HPL index respondents with major functional disabilities are
placed in the worst-health category regardless of prognosis or pathology.
This value judgment was based on the belief that such people were in the
worst health because they could not effectively perform basic activities of
daily living. This judgment is becoming widely accepted and is reflected
in the development of many scales of functional disability (Bergner et al.,
1976; Katz et al., 1971; Kohn and White, 1976), but it does not reflect the
prognostic significance, for example, of cancer.

Another decision made by HPL investigators was that in the index, all
chronic conditions would be given equal weight. Clearly, various chronic
conditions are not all equal in terms of prognosis or level of disability or
discomfort; moreover, the ranking of conditions poses considerable problems and is frequently controversial. In some indices, for example, Kisch
and colleagues (1969), weights are given for various conditions but no
rationale is provided for the weighting system. In other indices, such as
the Sickness Impact Profile (Carter et al., 1976), elaborate scaling systems
using hundreds of judges have been devised. Items have then been successfully ranked although disagreements among judges are still observed. In
the absence of a clear consensus for ranking chronic conditions, the HPL
investigators made a judgment to weight all conditions equally. In this
respect, further refinement of the HPL physical health status scale may be
in order.

Mental health or psychological well-being was determined largely from
several true–false questionnaire items designed to measure ego resiliency,
the presence of neurotic traits, and a sense of alienation or isolation known
as *anomie* (McCloskey and Schaar, 1965). Respondents also reported
whether they had suffered from emotional or mental illness and whether
they had visited a professional person for help with a mental or emotional

problem. Other questions elicited self-evaluations of general happiness, depression, restlessness, and other feeling states. The questionnaire incorporated items from the Bradburn-Caplovitz index of positive and negative feelings (Bradburn and Caplovitz, 1965). The HPL index, however, differs from the Bradburn-Caplovitz in omitting one item, "feeling proud because someone complimented you on something you had done"; also, it allows a longer period of time during which the feelings in question may have been experienced than the one specified in the Bradburn-Caplovitz study. Though the HPL index thus cannot strictly be considered validated by previous work done with the Bradburn-Caplovitz scale, it does apparently measure the same psychological dimension as that identified by the psychiatric ratings done in the Midtown Manhattan Study (Berkman, 1971a, b).

As an indication of social well-being, information was collected on the extent to which each individual was engaged in the social milieu of Alameda County. This included ascertaining whether a person lived with his or her family, and whether happily or not; the number of relatives and close friends, and the strength of connection with them; whether employed or not and other aspects of occupational adjustment; and the degree of relationship maintained with social and community organizations, such as in church, fraternal, union, and political groups. Social well-being constitutes one of the three dimensions of health in the WHO definition and was measured as such in the 1965 survey.

Selected items from the questionnaire pertaining to social well-being were also assembled into a Social Network Index. The latter constitutes one of the two components of life-style examined in this work with regard to their relationship to physical health and mortality. The other component of life-style to be explored consists of certain habits of daily life, including cigarette smoking, alcohol consumption, eating patterns, and level of physical activity.

The questionnaire also provided information about biologic factors such as age, height, and weight; use of medical care services; and demographic items such as race, sex, nativity, ethnicity, area of residence, and family status.

Thus items indicating physical, mental, and social well-being, items describing "ways of living" such as health practices and social networks, and certain demographic variables comprised the data from the Human Population Laboratory survey of Alameda County. The questionnaire, called "Health and Ways of Living," was 23 pages long and took the respondent about an hour to complete.

In order to assess health in relation to "ways of living," it was necessary to develop indices of variables being studied. Specifically for the analyses reported in this volume, the indices used are summary measures of physical health, health practices, and social networks. Brief descriptions of the latter two indices along with references to more detailed information appear in the following paragraphs.

When the Human Population Laboratory was getting under way, the idea was gradually being accepted that certain common personal habits such as cigarette smoking, alcohol consumption, physical exercise, eating regularly, and getting adequate amounts of sleep could affect physical health. There was, however, little solid evidence to support that idea except in the case of cigarette smoking. Items concerning a set of seven such habits were thus placed in the HPL questionnaire to comprise an index of health practices (Belloc and Breslow, 1972; Belloc et al., 1971).

1. "How many hours of sleep do you usually get a night?"
2. "How often do you eat breakfast?"
3. "How often do you eat in between your regular meals?"
4. "How often do you drink wine, beer, or liquor?"
5. "Have you ever smoked cigarettes regularly?" and "Do you smoke cigarettes at the present time?"
6. "Here is a list of active things that people do in their free time. How often do you do any of these things?" ("active sports," "swimming or taking long walks," "hunting or fishing," "doing physical exercises," "working in the garden")
7. "How tall are you?" and "How much do you weigh?"

In the construction of the index, one point was credited for each of the following answers: usual hours of sleep 7 or 8; eat breakfast almost every day; eat between meals only once in a while, rarely, or never; weight within the range of 5 percent under and 19.99 percent over the desirable standard for weight for men, or not more than 9.99 percent over for women; often or sometimes engage in active sports, swim, or take long walks, or often garden or do physical exercises; drink not more than four drinks at a time; never smoked cigarettes.

Previous reports from the Human Population Laboratory have dealt with all seven of these habits and their relationship to health and to mortality during the entire adult life span. In this monograph we consider in greater detail only five of these habits and their relationship to mortality and health status trends among persons 30–69 years of age over a 9-year follow-up period.

As noted previously, items concerning engagement with each person's social milieu were designed to provide a measure of social well-being, the third dimension of health in the WHO definition. Using some of the same items it was possible to construct a Social Network Index of social connections. Measures of marital status, contacts with extended family and close friends, church membership, and other group affiliations were combined to form the Social Network Index.

Two questions pertained to marital status: (1) "Have you ever been married?", and if so, (2) "Are you now married, separated, divorced, or widowed?" For the Social Network Index, respondents were categorized as being currently married or unmarried. Unmarried respondents could be single, separated, widowed, or divorced. Three questions delineated a second type of social contact: (1) "How many close friends do you have? (people that you feel at ease with, can talk to about private matters, and can call on for help)"; (2) "How many relatives do you have that you feel close to?"; and (3) "How many of these friends or relatives do you see at least once a month?" Responses to these items were rated on a 5-point scale: (1) None; (2) one or two; (3) three to five; (4) six to nine; and (5) ten or more. Respondents indicated belonging to a church by checking the appropriate box following the question: "Do you belong to any of these kinds of groups?" Respondents showed other group activities by checking yes or no to "a social or recreational group?"; "a labor union, commercial group, or professional association?"; "a group concerned with children (such as PTA or Boy Scout group)?"; "a group concerned with community betterment, charity, or service?"; "any other group?"

The Social Network Index summarizes not only the absolute number of social ties but also the degree of intimacy potentially provided by each source of contact. Thus the intimate contacts of marriage and contact with close friends and relatives are weighted more heavily than church affiliations and group memberships. Four networks categories were developed to reflect differences in type and extent of social contact (Berkman, 1977). The procedure by which this index was developed is explained more fully in Chapter 4.

The 1974 study

In 1974, The Human Population Laboratory conducted another study, with three major objectives:

1. To measure individual levels of physical, mental, and social well-being and ways of living again among the surviving respondents of the 1965 study after an interval of 9 years (the 1974 Panel Study)
2. To ascertain the completeness of the death clearance procedures, which had been ongoing since 1965

3. To gather information from a random sample of adults in Alameda County in 1974 in order to examine community changes in health and ways of living that had occurred between 1965 and 1974 (the 1974 HPL Survey).

The 1974 follow-up, called the Panel Study, was longitudinal in nature. It required that each surviving respondent who had supplied data in 1965 be contacted again, regardless of current location. Fieldwork for this follow-up study began in late 1973 and continued until October 1974. Procedures included initial interviewer contact at each address, enumeration of the household, and placement of appropriate questionnaires with each eligible person—that is, all 1965 respondents who could be found. Subsequently, the HPL staff initiated a record file for each household and each potential respondent. Failure to respond to the questionnaire triggered a sequential recovery effort that included, at 7-day intervals: a postcard reminder, a second questionnaire mailing, a certified letter reminder, and a telephone reminder. Finally, nonresponding persons were referred to the field staff for interviewer call-back to the household.

It was anticipated that, after an interval of 9 years, the longitudinal sample would have undergone substantial dispersion and attrition through residential mobility as well as a permanent loss by death. Death clearance during 1965 and subsequent years established that nearly 10 percent of the original 6928 respondents had died by 1974. Field operations revealed that another 59 percent of the 1965 study population had moved from their 1965 addresses. In order to locate these missing respondents an elaborate tracing procedure was developed and applied, involving contacts with a great variety of persons, institutions, and government agencies. Ultimately, this effort was reasonably successful, as Figure 2-3 shows. Geographic dispersion of 1965 respondents had taken place throughout California and to 43 other states and 20 foreign countries. Sixty percent of the movers, however, were still living within the greater San Francisco Bay area; only 15 percent had left California. Approximately 4 percent were found living overseas. Enumerators attempted to contact those still living in the nearby area, and most other former respondents were contacted by mail. An analysis of mobility among respondents to an HPL pilot study has also been reported by Carrington (1970). Perhaps the best indication of the effectiveness of the tracing procedure is that of the original 6928 respondents in 1965 who were presumably still living, only 272 could not be located in 1974. From Figure 2-3 it can also be seen that 4864 of the original 1965 respondents, 78 percent of those thought to be alive in 1974, answered the 1974 questionnaire and thereby became mem-

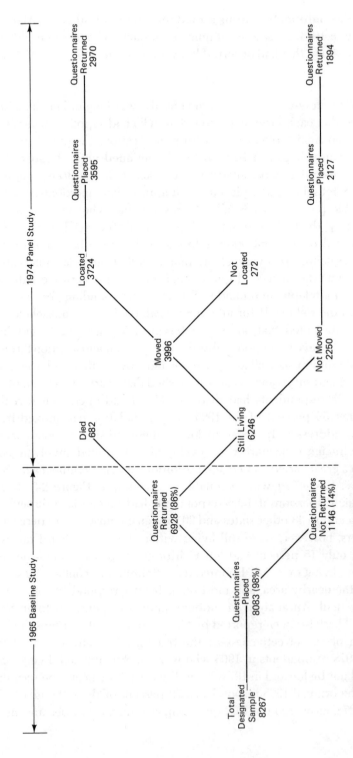

Fig. 2-3. Human Population Laboratory samples 1965–1974.

bers of the Panel Study. Bias introduced by panel attrition is discussed in Chapter 5.

The 1974 Panel Study questionnaire paralleled the 1965 baseline questionnaire in format and subject matter; most of the items asked in 1965 were repeated in the 1974 questionnaire. Dropped from the questionnaire were some items not subject to change, such as questions about the respondent's childhood; items with low reliability; and a few items found in analysis of the baseline data to be associated weakly or not at all with the major variables.

In addition to the items repeated from the 1964 questionnaire, two major new sets of items and several individual items were added to the 1974 survey. The two new sets focused on (1) stressful events, based on the Holmes and Rahe "Social Readjustment Rating Scale" (1967), that occurred in the respondent's life between 1965 and 1974; and (2) respondent's use of health care services including visits to a doctor, drug-utilization patterns, and use of screening and diagnostic services.

In the interim between the 1965 and 1974 surveys, the Human Population Laboratory collected mortality data on those who had died. A computer matching with the California Death Registry led to the records of those people who died within the state (Belloc and Arellano, 1973). Respondents were matched with death records on 3 primary items: the first four characters of the surname, sex, and color (white or nonwhite). Those records that matched on the 3 primary items were then compared on 10 secondary items including remaining characters from the surname; characters from first name and middle initial; month, day, and year of birth; and initial letter of birthplace. In the matching process, each of the secondary matching items was valued and weighted equally. The computer program printed out all pairs of records for which a score equal to or greater than a specified threshold value was attained. These printed linked records were then inspected visually; if judged to be possible matches, the original survey data were compared with the death certificate for ultimate verification.

For those who neither responded to the follow-up survey nor appeared in the California death clearance, out-of-state certificates were sought. If the 1974 follow-up survey indicated that an individual had died in a particular state, death clearance was sought from that state. Also, if an individual who could not be located in the follow-up survey was over 55 years of age and born out of state, an attempt was made to obtain death information from his or her state of birth.

In this manner, 682 death certificates were located for the 9-year period, 1965 to 1974. As previously mentioned, only 272 individuals or 4 percent of the sample were lost to follow-up. Those lost to follow-up did not differ markedly from the sample as a whole on the health measures in the 1965 survey. The collection of mortality data therefore seems to be fairly complete and unbiased.

The main purpose of the 1974 survey—to be distinguished from the 1974 Panel Study, just described—was to gather information on changes that had occurred during the 9-year period, 1965–1974, in the population's health status and health practices, and in social factors that might affect health status. The 1974 survey also sought information on utilization of health care services, perceived needs for services, and the extent to which the existing delivery systems met these needs.

The 1974 survey covered a sample of adults living in Alameda County that year, based on an area probability sample of housing units. It started with a subsample (50%) of the housing units used in the 1965 survey and added housing units created during the 9-year period in the same proportion as the 1965 housing unit sample. Although the sampling plan was less efficient than a newly constructed random sample of county residents, it had the advantage of low cost because it used the stable members of the panel and the addresses previously randomly drawn for the new occupants of the old dwellings. For reasons of cost and manageability, the 1974 sample was about half the size of that used in 1965.

The 1974 survey contained 4209 people in the total designated sample. Questionnaires were placed for 3868 and returned for 3121 persons, as seen in Table 2-7. Individuals selected for the 1974 survey received one of two questionnaire forms. A 28-page survey form containing those items relevant to the cross-sectional aspects of the study and emphasizing utilization and evaluation of health care delivery systems went to all persons who had not been respondents in the 1965 study. A 36-page combination form, containing items from both the longitudinal 1974 Panel Study and the cross-sectional 1974 survey, went to those 1965 respondents who were designated for inclusion in both the panel and survey samples. In both cases, questionnaire format and content were very similar to the original 1965 questionnaire, previously described.

Table 2-7. 1974 HPL survey questionnaire returns

Activity	Total 1974 survey		1974 survey only		Both 1965 and 1974 surveys	
	N	%	N	%	N	%
Questionnaire placed	3868	100.0	2938	100.0	930	100
Questionnaire returned	3121	80.7	2281	77.6	840	90.3

The evaluation of data: reliability and validity

A major problem area in survey research is the reliability and validity of collected data. The Human Population Laboratory has, therefore, made several efforts to examine the validity and reliability of the data through subsampling, resurveying, and gathering information from independent sources.

The major reliability studies were (1) a pilot study in 1961, followed up in 1964 (Meltzer and Hochstim, 1970); and (2) a random sample of 1530 adults in Alameda County who in 1968 filled out a shorter version of the baseline questionnaire and then filled out essentially the same form 1 to 2 weeks later (Hochstim and Renne, 1971). In those studies, which permitted assessment of the extent to which responses change over time, a reliable indicator was defined as one that consistently yields the same value as long as the particular condition being measured remains unchanged and changes its value only when the particular condition changes.

Table 2-8 shows the reliability of responses to seven demographic questions, theoretically invariable, asked of the same sample both in 1961 and 1964. As might be expected, the answers were quite stable: only 30 of a total of 2381 answers changed—an average of one percent. Also, relatively few people would be expected to change their marital status during a 3-year interval, and Table 2-9 reveals that 241 of 265 respondents, or 91 percent, gave identical answers in the two surveys. All but 1 of the 24 people who gave different answers could have been (and presumably were) reporting a true change.

In another study of reliability, a short period (2 weeks) between two surveys was assumed to preclude substantial real change. Different re-

Table 2-8. Consistency of responses to selected questions

Question	No. who answered both times	Percentage who answered consistently
Sex	265	100
Race	408	99
Born in United States	400	99
Father born in United States	392	98
Mother born in United States	398	98
Father deceased by 1961	257	100
Mother deceased by 1961	261	99

From Hochstim, J.R.: Health and Ways of Living: The Alameda County Population Laboratory. In Kessler, I.J., Levin, M.L. (eds.): *The Community as an Epidemiological Laboratory*. Baltimore, Johns Hopkins University Press, 1970, p. 162.

Table 2-9. Consistency of responses on marital status pilot study sample, 1961–1964

Marital status in 1964	Marital status in 1961				
	Married	Widowed	Divorced	Separated	Never married
Total	217	17	9	4	18
Married	212[a]	3	3	0	9
Widowed	3	14	0	1	0
Divorced	1	0	5	2	0
Separated	1	0	0	1	0
Never married	0	0	1	0	9

[a]Responses identical on both surveys.

From Hochstim, J.R.: Health and Ways of Living: The Alameda County Population Laboratory. In Kessler, I.J., Levin, M.L. (eds.): *The Community as an Epidemiological Laboratory*, Baltimore, Johns Hopkins University Press, 1970, p. 162.

sponses to the same question would indicate unreliability of response. The sample consisted of the adults living in approximately 1000 Alameda County households. All the procedures were as much like those used in the 1965 survey as possible. An enumerator left a self-administered questionnaire for each adult in the household. On the following day the enumerator returned to pick up the completed questionnaires, explaining at that time that the second part of the questionnaire would be sent by mail and that it would be picked up one week later. The second part was essentially a duplicate of the first part. Eighty-four percent of the persons contacted filled in both questionnaires.

Most of the questionnaire items fell into five subject areas, the first two predominantly objective, and the last three predominantly subjective in nature: (1) demographic questions; (2) chronic conditions; (3) symptoms or ailments; (4) marital satisfaction; and (5) psychological indices. A large proportion of the responses seemed reliable. Practically all (98%) of the respondents answered at least 80 percent of the items identically on both surveys, including 74 percent who answered at least 90 percent of the items identically. Only 2 percent did so in as few as 70–79 percent of the items. Reliability was highest for the more objective questions, and lowest where mood or attitude appeared as a strong factor.

In order to discount the agreement between items that can be attributed to chance, an index of reliability was developed: the excess of the observed agreement over the agreement to be expected on the basis of the marginal distribution, as a percentage of the maximum possible value of the excess. Table 2-10 shows that for the set of 35 questions on physical health, the index of reliability is 82. This means that the observed agreement exceeded the agreement expected on the basis of chance by four-fifths as much as theoretically possible, given the marginal distributions of the two sets of responses. Chronic conditions were reported with a reliability index value of 88, whereas the psychological and marital satisfaction items showed lower reliability index values, ranging from 64 to 74. This progression in consistency of response corresponds roughly to the degree of objectivity involved in questionnaire responses, indicating that reliability is as much a function of the content of the question as it is an attribute of respondents or questionnaire format. Of further interest was the fact that the direction of change definitely tended toward a better rather than a poorer image of the respondent.

Of the total number of responses to 60 dichotomous items, 94 percent remained on the same favorable or unfavorable side. One-fourth of the initially unfavorable responses changed, while only 3 percent of the favorable responses changed.

Several attempts were also made to test the validity of answers to specific questions. For example, the 1965 study queried respondents as to whether they had voted in the 1964 presidential election, and, if they had, whether they had voted in Alameda County. The official county voting

Table 2-10. Index of reliability by subject matter for 60 dichotomous items

| Type of item | No. of items | No. of responses | Percentage in agreement | | | Index of reliability[b] $\dfrac{(A) - (B)}{(C) - (B)}$ |
			Obser-ved (A)	Expec-ted[a] (B)	Maxi-mum[a] (C)	
All items	60	87,858	94	73	99	79
Physical health	35	53,225	96	85	99	82
Disabilities	5	7,610	96	82	99	80
Chronic conditions	16	24,373	99	92	100	88
Impairments	3	4,571	98	93	99	82
Symptoms	11	16,671	93	75	98	79
Psychological	19	28,067	89	61	98	76
Anomy	9	13,263	86	52	98	74
Isolation/depression	9	13,333	92	76	98	69
Happiness	1	1,471	92	81	98	64
Marital satisfaction	6	6,566	94	80	99	72

[a]Given the two marginal distributions.

[b]Index values were calculated from the *numbers* observed, expected, and so on, so in many cases they are more accurate than the values one would obtain using the rounded percentages in the tables.

From Hochstim, J.R., Renne, K.S.: Reliability of response in a sociomedical population study. *Public Opinion Quarterly* 35:69–79, 1971.

records verified the respondent's answer in 94 percent of a subsample checked (Hochstim, 1970).

A pilot study queried women as to whether they had ever had a Papanicolaou test for cervical cancer or, if not, whether they had ever received a pelvic examination. Those who reported either the test or the examination were asked to name the physician or hospital involved, providing an opportunity to check the validity of their answer. In 91 percent of the cases, the medical facility had some record of the respondent; and in 84 percent the questionnaire response was confirmed (Hochstim and Breslow, 1963).

In the 1965 study, health conditions reported on the questionnaires were compared with the medical records for the 902 respondents who were members of the Kaiser Foundation Health Plan. Of 902 respondents, 739 had received either the multiphasic screening examination or some other general physical examination during 1963–1965. Physicians reviewed the Kaiser records and attempted to rate each person in the HPL study who had such a record on certain variables used in the analysis of the survey data, working without knowledge of the person's questionnaire responses. Physical health as ascertained in the 1965 survey would obviously be difficult to validate from medical records. For example, the survey information about minor disability was based on such questions as this: "Have you had to cut down or stop any other activity (meaning other than work) you used to do because of some illness or injury? For example, you have to 'take it easy,' or cut out some sport, or find you can't spend as many hours gardening as you used to." Medical records often fail to supply information of this kind. Nevertheless, physician raters estimated each person's physical health classification on the HPL spectrum from the medical records as best they could. A cross-classification of survey ratings on the HPL Physical Health Index and the medical records rating appears in Table 2-11, where the unit is a person rather than a condition. A total of 361 persons, or 49 percent, received the identical rating on the basis of Kaiser records as they did from the questionnaire data. An additional 38 percent of the ratings agreed within one category.

Another way to express the degree of agreement between the survey and medical records is by an index of agreement—that is, the excess of the observed agreement over the agreement expected by chance, expressed as a percentage of the maximum possible value of the excess, given the two marginal distributions. As seen in Table 2-12, abstracts of medical records "confirmed" 92 and 97 percent of their "No's." The index of agreement for the whole set of questions was 37; that is, the observed agreement was 37 percent better than could be expected on the basis of the marginal distributions of the two sets of questionnaires. The 14 ques-

Table 2-11. Physical Health Spectrum: survey ratings and abstractor's ratings, according to number of respondents, for the medical record check sample

Survey ratings	All respondents	Abstractor's rating			
		A	B	C	D
All respondents	739	29	315	189	206
A Disabilities[a]	92	19	55	13	5
B Chronic conditions or impairments but no disability	241	10	166	34	31
C Symptoms only	222	—	54	87	81
D No problem	184	—	40	55	89

[a]Disabilities of less than 6 months' duration are excluded.

From Meltzer, J.W., Hochstim, J.R.: Reliability and validity of survey data on physical health. *Public Health Reports* 85:1075–1086, 1970.

tions on chronic illness agreed better with the medical records than did the three other types of complaints. Over half (54 percent) of the chronic conditions reported in the survey were also noted in the record, and the index of agreement for the questions on chronic conditions is 52.

These comparisons, of course, do not constitute true measures of validity. To the extent that the two records agree, however, one may presume that both are valid. When they disagree, either record may be in error or incomplete, or they may simply contain different kinds of information, collected for different purposes on different occasions.

Table 2-12. Index of agreement between survey data and medical record data for medical record check sample: type of complaint

Type of complaint	Total No. of responses	Index of agreement	Percentage of record items in agreement with survey response		
			All	Yes	No
All types	24,301	37	92	33	97
Disabilities[a]	3,693	45	95	16	99
Chronic conditions	10,322	52	96	54	98
Impairments	2,207	31	96	28	98
Symptoms	8,079	28	84	28	93

[a]Disabilities of less than 6 months' duration are excluded.

From Meltzer, J.W., Hochstim, J.R.: Reliability and validity of survey data on physical health. *Public Health Report* 85:1075–1086, 1970.

Although there has been considerable work on the question of validity of the Human Population Laboratory physical health items, validation of psychological and social items has received less effort. This has been true in part because of the inherent difficulty of validating such items.

Focus of the monograph

The original objectives of the Human Population Laboratory, as stated previously, were to develop measures of physical, mental, and social well-being, to examine whether and how they were interrelated, and to determine the relationship of health to ways of living and demographic characteristics. As analysis of the data commenced, however, the third objective attracted major attention. The relationship of common daily behaviors (called "health practices"), such as physical activity, cigarette smoking, and alcohol consumption, to physical health status and mortality became relatively more prominent in the study. Along with other compelling evidence linking tobacco and alcohol use to health status, this work helped establish the importance of disease prevention through behavioral changes. Though the work on health practices is subject to methodological criticisms, it seems important for two reasons:

1. It suggests that certain behaviors have generalized health, rather than just specific disease, consequences.
2. It identifies a series of common behaviors rather than rare exposures or experiences that might, because of their distribution in the population, play an important role in determining the health status of large populations.

Research extending over several decades on cigarette smoking, physical activity, alcohol consumption, and certain dietary patterns has indicated that these practices are associated with specific disease entities, for example, cigarette smoking with lung cancer, and alcohol with cirrhosis of liver. Recent studies show that most of these same practices are also associated, though not as strongly, with other diseases. Smoking is a risk factor in coronary heart disease, many types of cancer, and respiratory illnesses (U.S., D.H.E.W., 1979; WHO, 1975). Alcohol consumption appears to promote certain kinds of tumor growth, especially in combination with tobacco (Rothman, 1975; Rothman and Keller, 1972; Wynder and Bross, 1957) and may harm the fetus in pregnant women (Ouellette et al., 1977; Streissguth, 1978). Thus although some of these behaviors undoubtedly play a strong role in specific diseases, it now appears that they may also influence health in a more general way.

Previous work from the Human Population Laboratory had not fully sorted out the independent effects of the seven health practices from their possibly confounding effects on one another. Whether physical activity is related to physical health status independently of obesity, for example, or through its association with that variable was not clear. The HPL survey had covered many kinds of behavior, although detailed information in some areas such as diet was lacking.

Important as it was to assess the independent effects of the health practices, it was equally appropriate to assess their joint contribution. Because there were several moderately positive correlations among the health practices, their cumulative effect might be less than additive. On the other hand, it was also plausible that they could have synergistic effects. In either case, measuring their effects as a whole and in various combinations would be relevant.

There is another reason to examine the health practices jointly: they may reflect some underlying common pattern of living such as moderation and regularity. It seemed desirable to gain a better understanding of how the health practices are related to one another and to other variables. Therefore, while analyzing the impact of the practices on physical health, we also wanted to examine the interrelationships of these variables and their associations with other psychological, social, and environmental variables.

The search for ways of life beyond the health practices that might have a broad health impact disclosed evidence in the HPL data for a second set of factors, very different from the health practices. This set consisted of items indicating degree to which people maintain social and community ties, that is, a social network. Although there is not much epidemiologic research on these factors, data concerning relocation, urbanization, widowhood, mobility, and migration increasingly suggest that different and changing social environments are associated with a wide range of diseases. These data support, albeit indirectly, the idea that social connections may be significant for health.

Several investigators, most notably John Cassel (1974, 1976; Cassel and Tyroler, 1961), Aaron Antonovsky (1972, 1973, 1976, 1979), and S. Leonard Syme (1974; Syme and Torfs, 1978), have made important theoretical contributions that have laid the groundwork for research in this area. They have each proposed that social and community ties may have an impact on health status by influencing physiological mechanisms, most likely neural, hormonal, or immunologic control systems, which in turn influence host susceptibility to a wide variety of diseases.

We hypothesized that the kinds and degrees of social ties an individual maintained with others might be related to vulnerability to disease in general. With the intent of measuring social well-being, the 1965 HPL survey had included a range of questions concerning respondent's degree of connectedness with his social network. These questions proved adequate for the purpose of measuring social ties.

A secondary objective of this part of the analysis was to understand the relationship between social networks and other social and psychological factors. Clearly, the kinds of social relationships an individual develops are influenced by his or her social circumstances and psychological characteristics. For instance, it is easy to conceive of social conditions such as poverty, mobility, and migration, as well as psychological states such as depression, alienation, and low self-esteem, which might have profound influences on social network development. Although a comprehensive analysis of the interactions among these factors would make another book, we believed that it would be useful in the present work to gain some grasp of them, for three reasons. First, it is possible that these factors could seriously confound the relationship of health to social network variables by either obscuring an association or spuriously making one appear. Thus our analyses reflect a desire to assess the independent effect of social networks on risk of dying or decline in physical health status over the 9-year follow-up period. Second, we wished to examine any factors that might mediate such a relationship, particularly psychological ones. Third, we wanted to understand how social networks and health practices are related to other psychosocial variables so that effective interventions in this area can eventually be developed.

The unraveling of associations between socioeconomic status and social networks, health practices, and mortality is obviously important. Because socioeconomic status is known to be associated with health status and many behavioral factors, we examined these variables carefully. Dimensions of mental well-being such as depression, alienation, and positive and negative feelings were also included in the analysis, because emotional and other psychological states may play some role in causing disease and in shaping certain behaviors.

The relationships among these variables are to be examined cross-sectionally from data collected in the 1965 survey. Thus no inferences can be drawn concerning the determinants of social networks or health practices. We can, however, assess the independent relationship of these variables to physical health and examine correlations with other psychological and social circumstances.

A word about the measurement of physical health status may be appropriate at this point. In the first two chapters we have emphasized that physical health status should be conceptualized in a non-disease-specific way as well as in traditional disease-specific terms. Research along these lines has led to the development of several health indices (Bergner et al., 1976; Brodman et al., 1949; Elinson, 1976). The Human Population Laboratory's own measure of physical health is another contribution to this literature (Belloc et al., 1971). After thus emphasizing the importance of morbidity, we still concentrate in this monograph on mortality. An explanation is in order.

We chose "mortality from all causes" as the major dependent variable for several reasons. First, death is not subject to the bias of self-report, measurement error, or misclassification of disease status. Moreover, the study of total mortality is not subject to the difficulties inherent in cause-of-death classifications based on death certificates. Finally, the Human Population Laboratory mortality follow-up of 9 years, from 1965 to 1974, coupled with responses to the 1965 survey, provides a strong cohort or longitudinal study design. Some pitfalls and biases frequently encountered in cross-sectional or retrospective study designs are avoided.

The use of mortality data, however, carried several limitations. First, people who died during the 9-year follow-up period might have been diseased at the time of the survey. The relationship among social networks and health practices and mortality could therefore have resulted because people who were ill at the time of the survey were physically unable to maintain certain health-promoting behaviors or social contacts; this possible reversal of the hypothesized causal chain will be explored in Chapters 3, 4, and 5.

The second limitation of these data also emerges from the possible association between mortality and prior illness. Our hypothesis that social and behavioral factors influence susceptibility to disease in general may imply that these factors affect the incidence of disease. Mortality data such as those used in our analyses, however, do not reveal whether the risk factors influence disease incidence per se or the survival time between onset of disease and death. In either case, host resistance may be implicated, but from mortality data alone we do not know where along the spectrum of disease occurrence and course the social and behavioral factors have their greatest impact.

Because we wanted to gain some insight into this problem, we decided to supplement our mortality analyses with some data on morbidity. For this purpose James Wiley and Terry Camacho examined the impact of social networks and health practices as measured in 1965 on changes in morbidity between 1965 and 1974, when the follow-up survey was conducted. This analysis is reported in Chapter 6.

The aim of this monograph, then, is to examine whether two sets of factors—social networks and common daily behaviors—have generalized health consequences. Their relationship to physical health is assessed by all-cause mortality and a general measure of morbidity. Ours is a cohort study, comparing initial responses to the 1965 survey with 9-year follow-up information on mortality and changes in morbidity.

References

Antonovsky A: Breakdown: a needed fourth step in the conceptual armamentarium of modern medicine. *Soc. Sci. Med.* 6:537–544, 1972.

Antonovsky A: The utility of the breakdown concept. *Soc. Sci. Med.* 7:605–612, 1973.

Antonovsky A: Conceptual and methodological problems in the study of resistance resources and stressful life events, in Dohrenwend B, Dohrenwend B (eds): *Stressful Life Events: Their Nature and Consequences.* New York, John Wiley & Sons, 1976, pp. 245–258.

Antonovsky A: *Health, Stress, and Coping.* Chicago, Jossey-Bass, 1979.

Balinsky W, Berger R: A review of the research on General Health Status Indexes. *Med. Care* 13(4):283–293, 1975.

Belloc N, Arellano M: Computer record linkage on a survey population. *Health Serv. Rep.* 88(4):344–350, 1973.

Belloc, NB, Breslow L, Hochstim JR: Measurement of physical health in a general population survey. *Am. J. Epidemiol.* 93(5):328–336, 1971.

Belloc NB, Breslow L: Relationship of physical health status and health practices. *Prev. Med.* 13:409–421, 1972.

Bergner M, Bobbitt R, Kressel S, et al.: The sickness impact profile: conceptual formulation and methodology for the development of a health status measure. *Int. J. Health Serv.* 6(3):393–415, 1976.

Berkman LF: *Social Networks, Host Resistance, and Mortality: a Follow-up Study of Alameda County Residents,* doctoral thesis, University of California, Berkeley, 1977.

Berkman P: Life stress and psychological well-being: a replication of Langner's analysis in the Midtown Manhattan Study. *J. Health Soc. Behav.* 12:35–45, 1971a.

Berkman PL: Measurement of mental health in a general population survey. *Am. J. Epidemiol.* 94(2):105–111, 1971b.

Bradburn NM, Caplovitz D: *Reports on Happiness: A Pilot Study of Behavior Related to Mental Health.* Chicago, Aldine, 1965.

Breslow L: A quantitative approach to the World Health Organization definition of health: physical, mental and social well-being. *Int. J. Epidemiol.* 1:347–355, 1972.

Breslow L, Hochstim JR: Socio-cultural aspects of cervical cytology in Alameda County, California. *Public Health Rep.* 79:107–112, 1964.

Brodman K, Erdmann A, Lorge L, et al.: The Cornell Medical Index. An adjunct to medical interview. *J. A. M. A.* 140:530–534, 1949.

California State Dept. of Public Health: *Alameda County Population 1965.* April 1966.

Carrington RA: Analysis of mobility and change in a longitudinal sample. *Public Health Rep.* 85:49–58, 1970.

Carter WB, Bobbitt R, Bergner M, Gilson B: Validation of an interval scaling: the Sickness Impact Profile. *Health Serv. Res.* 11(4):516–528, 1976.

Cassel J: Psychosocial processes and "stress": theoretical formulation. *Int. J. Health Serv.* 4(3):471–482, 1974.

Cassel J: The contribution of the social environment to host resistance. *Am. J. Epidemiol.* 104(2):107–123, 1976.

Cassel J, Tyroler HA: Epidemiological studies of culture change. Health status and recency of industrialization. *Arch. Environ. Health* 3:25–33, 1961.

Elinson J (ed): Sociomedical health indicators. *Int. J. Health Serv.* (Special issue) 6(3):377–538, 1976.

Goldsmith S: The status of health status indicators. *Health Serv. Rep.* 87(3):212–220, 1972.

Hochstim JR: *Comparison of Three Information-Gathering Strategies in a Population Study of Sociomedical Variables.* Berkeley, California State Dept. of Public Health, 1962.

Hochstim JR: A critical comparison of three strategies of collecting data from households. *J. Amer. Statistics Assoc.* 62:976–989, 1967.

Hochstim JR: Health and ways of living: the Alameda County Population Laboratory, in Kessler IJ, Levin ML (eds): *The Community as an Epidemiological Laboratory.* Baltimore, Johns Hopkins University Press, 1970, pp. 149–176.

Hochstim JR, Breslow L: *Cervical Cytology in Alameda County.* Berkeley, California State Dept. of Public Health, January 1963.

Hochstim JR, Athanasopoulos DA, Larkins JH: Poverty area under the microscope. *Am. J. Public Health* 58:1815–1827, 1968.

Hochstim JR, Athanasopoulos DA: Personal follow-up in a mail survey: its contribution and its cost. *Public Opinion Q.* 34:69–81, 1970.

Hochstim JR, Renne KS: Reliability of response in a sociomedical population study. *Public Opinion Q.* 35:69–79, 1971.

Holmes TH, Rahe RH: The social readjustment rating scale. *J. Psychosom. Res.* 11:213–218, 1967.

Katz S, Akpom CA, Papsidero JA, Weiss ST: A measure of health status (Need, use of services, expectations, barriers), in Sackett DL, Baskin MS (eds): *Methods of Health Care Evaluation.* Hamilton, Ont., McMaster University, 1971, chap. 3.

Kisch A, Kovner J, Harris L, Kline G: A new proxy measure for health status. *Health Serv. Res.* 4:223–230, 1969.

Kohn R, White KL (eds): *Health Care: An International Study. Report of the World Health Organization/International Collaborative Study of Medical Care Utilization.* London, Oxford University Press, 1976.

McCloskey H, Schaar JH: Psychological dimensions of anomy. *Am. Sociol. Rev.* 30:14–40, 1965.

Meltzer JW, Hochstim JR: Reliability and validity of survey data on physical health. *Public Health Rep.* 85:1075–1086, 1970.

Ouellette EM, Rosett HL, Rosman NP, et al.: Adverse effects on offspring of maternal alcohol abuse during pregnancy. *N. Engl. J. Med.* 297:528–530, 1977.

Rothman KJ: Alcohol, in Fraumeni JF (ed): *Persons at High Risk of Cancer: An Approach to Cancer Etiology and Control.* New York, Academic Press, 1975, pp. 139–150.

Rothman KJ, Keller AZ: The effect of joint exposure to alcohol and tobacco on
    risk of cancer of the mouth and pharynx. *J. Chron. Dis.* **25**:711–716, 1972.

Streissguth AP: Fetal alcohol syndrome: an epidemiologic perspective. *Am. J.
    Epidemiol.* **107**(6):467–478, 1978.

Syme SL: Behavioral factors associated with the etiology of disease: a social
    epidemiological perspective. *Am. J. Public Health* **64**:1043–1045, 1974.

Syme SL: Torfs CP: Epidemiologic research in hypertension: a critical appraisal.
    J. Hum. Stress **4**:43–48, 1978.

United States, Dept. of Health, Education and Welfare, Public Health Service:
    Smoking and Health. Washington, D.C., U.S. Government Printing Office,
    1979.

World Health Organization. Smoking and disease: the evidence reviewed. *WHO
    Chron.* **29**:402–408, 1975.

Wynder EL, Bross IJ: Aetiological factors in mouth cancer. *Br. Med. J.* 1:1137–1143,
    May 18, 1957.

3. Health practices and mortality risk

LISA F. BERKMAN   LESTER BRESLOW
DEBORAH WINGARD

In the last 20 years a vast body of evidence has accumulated indicating that certain common behaviors, particularly cigarette smoking, physical activity, and alcohol consumption, play a role in the development of disease. Since its inception, the Human Population Laboratory has had a strong commitment to conducting research in this area. Based on the cross-sectional data from the 1965 survey, Belloc and Breslow (1972) reported an association between physical health status and seven common health-related activities or characteristics: (1) physical activity, (2) cigarette smoking, (3) alcohol consumption, (4) obesity, (5) sleeping habits, (6) eating breakfast daily, and (7) snacking between meals. In subsequent work, they found these seven factors (which we will refer to as health practices for the sake of brevity) to be related to 6-year mortality risk (Belloc, 1973).

Studies of health practices

Findings from other population studies also illustrate the importance of some, although not all, of the health practices examined in the HPL survey. Data from Framingham reveal the relation of physical inactivity, obesity, and especially smoking to subsequent morbidity and mortality (Kannel, 1967). Analysis of information from more than one million adult men and women by the American Cancer Society indicates that lack of exercise, cigarette smoking, sleeping over 8 hours per night, being over-

weight, or losing 10 or more pounds in the last 5 years were each independently associated with increased mortality from coronary heart disease (CHD) and stroke (Hammond, 1964; Hammond and Garfinkel,
1969).

Several investigations of this matter have focused on unique population
groups, and findings from them may be less generalizable to the population as a whole than are large-scale community studies. For example,
Paffenbarger and his colleagues (1970, 1975, 1977, 1978) have reported on
the mortality experience of longshoremen employed in San Francisco in
1951. For this select group of men, energy output at work, cigarette
smoking, body weight for height, blood cholesterol, blood pressure, prior
heart disease, and glucose metabolism were determined during examinations in 1951 and subsequently. Cigarette smoking was related to mortality
from heart disease, cancer, chronic obstructive respiratory disease, and
pneumonia. Inactivity predicted fatal heart disease.

In another study, data on smoking, physical activity, and relative body
weight were obtained from male patients 30 to 64 years old, who had
experienced myocardial infarction at least 3 months previously and were
now attending Coronary Drug Project centers (1974, 1975). After 3 years,
only physical inactivity appeared independently related to mortality.
Later, both smoking and inactivity were related to increased mortality
whereas obesity was not.

Several investigators have explored the mortality experience of specific
religious groups. For example, Enstrom (1975) has shown that adult
Mormons in California between 1970 and 1972 experienced only one-half
to three-fourths the cancer death rate of other Californians. Active
Mormons had lower cancer rates than inactive Mormons. The strongly
Mormon state of Utah experienced the lowest mortality from cancer in
the country, about 70 percent of the U.S. rate. Lyon and his colleagues
(1976) reported similar findings between 1966 and 1970 in Utah. The
church's doctrine forbidding the use of tobacco, alcohol, coffee, and tea,
and recommending a certain diet was suggested as possibly contributing
to the low cancer rate. Data on Seventh-Day Adventists have likewise
indicated a link between life-style and cancer (Phillips, 1975), coronary
artery disease (Wynder et al., 1959), (Phillips et al., 1980), and respiratory
system disease (Lemon and Walden, 1966). It is difficult, however, to
separate the effects of health practices from other aspects of life-style
common among those belonging to such religions, for example, differing
social stresses and network systems.

Studies of health practices must include consideration of correlated
factors that may affect morbidity and mortality, particularly social and
cultural forces and personality characteristics that play a role in deter-

mining habits. For example, persons in lower classes tend to be more obese and also to smoke cigarettes more frequently (Khosla and Lowe, 1972). In the Tecumseh Community Health Study, Higgins et al. (1967) found that smokers differed from nonsmokers in that they were more likely to come from families where people smoked, to live in urban rather than rural areas, and to drink alcohol. Among men, smokers were more likely to have blue-collar jobs. Among women, on the other hand, smokers tend to be better educated and to have white-collar jobs. The concordance between smoking and alcohol consumption suggests that both may be influenced by some common factors. In a more recent study of the same Tecumseh population, Metzner et al. (1977a) studied 1144 adults to determine the effect of life stresses on health practices and health. Early childhood residential mobility was related to the presence of chronic conditions and nine risk factors (including obesity, smoking, and alcohol consumption) in adult women, but not in men.

The relationships between life changes or stresses, and health practices are becoming better understood. In a group of 34 Navy company commanders, Conway and co-workers (1981) found that on high-stress days, when commanders were training new recruits, there was more cigarette smoking and coffee drinking but less alcohol consumption. These general effects of stress appeared to reflect largely the behavior of only a few officers, suggesting important individual differences in the tendency to increase or decrease habitual substance consumption in response to varying levels of stress. Similar results have been reported by Lindenthal et al. (1972) with regard to smoking behavior. These investigators found a strong association between catastrophic events and increase of smoking, especially for the psychiatrically impaired. They suggest that smoking is one way some individuals try to cope with adverse events. Pearson (1974) has also reported that among nursing students good health practices declined with increasing numbers of significant life changes.

In addition to the data about such general health practices, a vast literature describes specific individual behaviors and their relationships to physical health status and mortality. This evidence will be reviewed briefly.

Physical activity

Physical activity has been studied extensively as a possible factor in coronary heart disease. In a comprehensive review of the literature, Froelicher (1976) concludes that physical inactivity has been demonstrated to be a risk factor for CHD, but not with the same high level of confidence as other risk factors: hypercholesterolemia, hypertension, and cigarette smoking.

From the Framingham Study of 5127 men and women, Kannel (1967) created a physical activity index by summing the products of weighted hours spent at various levels of physical activity in a usual 24-hour day, and he also rated activity indirectly by weight gain, vital capacity, and resting pulse rate. His analysis indicated that CHD and mortality are related to a sedentary life-style. Paffenbarger and Hale (1975) classified 6351 San Francisco longshoremen with respect to physical activity at work in 1951 as heavy, moderate, and light. Age-adjusted death rates for CHD over the next 22 years among those with heavy physical activity at work were 26.9 per 10,000 man-years; moderate, 46.3; and light, 49.0. The association was stronger for sudden than for delayed death (after one hour), and persisted when controlling for age, job changes, and five other risk factors including smoking and obesity.

In connection with each of the foregoing reports, it should be remembered that physical health status may influence activity level, both at home and on the job. For example, physical activity declines with severe injury or chronic illness. Paffenbarger and his colleagues considered this aspect of the problem by taking into account both original and more recent physical activity on the job, and years of exposure to each.

One may also examine this issue by studying physiological responses to exercise, such as heart rate changes with treadmill tests, and the differences between athletes and nonathletes with respect to blood pressure, resting heart rate, and recovery time. In Tecumseh, Michigan, Montoye (1975) found that those who exercised regularly tended to recover their normal heart rate quicker and had lower blood pressure. Athletes had lower resting heart rates, and obesity was associated with inactivity. Vigorous exercise of animals can produce myocardial hypertrophy, histologic changes, increase in coronary artery size, coronary collateral circulation, and improved cardiac performance (Froelicher, 1976).

Cigarette smoking

Cigarette smoking is probably the most extensively studied practice affecting health. Since 1964, Public Health Service reviews of smoking and health studies have repeatedly shown that cigarette smoking is related to overall mortality. The 1975 report of the surgeon general, *The Health Consequences of Smoking*, summarized the evidence indicating cigarette smoking to be an important factor in cancer, cardiovascular disease, and chronic respiratory disease (U.S., D.H.E.W., 1975). The World Health Organization came to similar conclusions in a 1975 review.

In one of the earliest studies, Doll and Hill (1964) in 1951 sent mail questionnaires about smoking habits to physicians in England. Although response to the survey was only 68 percent, mortality follow-up after 10 years was nearly complete. Death rates, standardized for age and for each sex, showed a strong association with smoking. Among men, the association prevailed for several causes of death, including lung cancer, chronic bronchitis, pulmonary tuberculosis, coronary disease without hypertension, and peptic ulcer; among women, it held only for lung cancer. Death rates increased with amount smoked and declined with years since quitting.

The American Cancer Society questionnaire survey of one million men and women from 25 different states likewise revealed that smokers have higher age-adjusted death rates, especially for certain causes of death such as emphysema and lung cancer (Hammond, 1966). During 4 years of follow-up, from 1959 to 1963, higher death rates were found among those who smoked large numbers of cigarettes, inhaled deeply, and started to smoke while young. Among those who had quit, death rates were lower with increasing number of years since smoking stopped.

The Dorn study of smoking and mortality among U.S. veterans disclosed after 8½ years of observation that cigarette smokers had 1.7 times the total death rate of nonsmokers (Kahn, 1966). Death rates increased with the number of cigarettes smoked and the length of time the individual had smoked.

In addition to studies of smoking and total mortality, other investigations have revealed the relationship of smoking to individual diseases (U.S., D.H.E.W., 1975). For instance, the Dorn study showed mortality ratios to be much higher for lung cancer (10.9) and emphysema (12.2) than for coronary heart disease (1.6). Even greater differences in these cause-specific relative risks were reported by Doll and Hill (1964). Whereas the relationship of cigarette smoking to many forms of cancer, chronic bronchitis, and emphysema has been established beyond reasonable doubt, its relationship to cardiovascular disease is not as clear. Cigarette smoking was associated with CHD among male blue-collar workers in Framingham, but not among white-collar workers or women (Haynes et al., 1980). Both the Framingham cohort (Gordon and Kannel, 1972) and a longitudinal study of former college students (Paffenbarger and Wing, 1971) showed an association between cigarette smoking and stroke. Several other morbidity and mortality studies of stroke, however —in Washington County, Maryland (Nomura et al., 1974), Chicago

(Ostfeld et al., 1974), and Hiroshima (Johnson et al., 1967)—revealed no relationship between stroke and cigarette smoking. On balance it appears that cigarette smoking is strongly associated with CHD and with lung diseases. The data are inconclusive with regard to stroke.

The synergistic effects of cigarette smoking combined with other risk factors seem to be remarkably strong. When combined with oral contraceptive use, asbestos exposures, alcohol consumption, or hypertension risk, relative risks of smoking are increased for nonfatal myocardial infarction (Rosenberg et al., 1980), and greatly increased for cancer of the oral cavity and lung (Rothman, 1975; Selikoff et al., 1968; Wynder and Bross, 1957).

Numerous animal and experimental studies also indicate the effect of cigarette smoking on longevity and physiological functions, and point to certain physiological mechanisms that may be involved (U.S., D.H.E.W., 1975). Carbon monoxide has been implicated in the development of atherosclerosis (Astrup, 1973), and nicotine induces several pharmacologic effects on the heart that may be responsible for increased rates of myocardial infarction and sudden death (Bellen et al., 1972; Greenspan et al., 1969; Levine, 1973; Ostfeld, 1980).

In considering the effect of smoking on humans, it is important to keep in mind that people's health may influence their smoking habits. A person with heart trouble or lung cancer may be told by a physician to stop smoking. A 4-year prospective study of more than 300,000 adult men conducted by the American Cancer Society showed ex-smokers to have a higher death rate than current smokers (Hammond, 1966). If the analysis controlled for health status at the time of the questionnaire, however, ex-smokers had lower death rates. The study also indicated that cigarette smokers in poor health often switched to brands containing low amounts of nicotine and tar.

Obesity

Obesity has long been associated with excessive morbidity and mortality. According to studies reviewed by Levinson (1977) and the U.S. Department of Health, Education and Welfare (1966), obesity carries increased risk of cardiovascular and pulmonary difficulties and of impaired carbohydrate metabolism. It aggravates other conditions such as hypertension, diabetes, and arthritis, and adds risk to surgery and pregnancy.

The dangers of obesity became especially evident after the Society of Actuaries published findings from the *Build and Blood Pressure Study* of 1959, covering the mortality experience of about 5 million people insured by 27 large life insurance companies in the United States and Canada from 1935 to 1953 (Metropolitan Life Insurance Company, 1959, 1960). The investigation demonstrated that obesity was associated with higher mortality. Men and women had an excess mortality of 13 and 9 percent, respectively, when 10 percent overweight; mortality jumped to 42 and 30 percent when men and women were 30 percent overweight. The higher death rates were chiefly caused by diseases of the heart and circulatory system (Metropolitan Life Insurance Company, 1959, 1960). On the basis of that study the Metropolitan Life Insurance Company revised its tables of desirable weights for height—that is, weights associated with lowest mortality among men and women over 25 years old having small, medium, and large frames (Metropolitan Life Insurance Company 1959, 1960). These "norms" have become a standard used by many physicians and in research projects to measure obesity.

Following the Build and Blood Pressure Study, several prospective morbidity and mortality studies included weight for height, skinfold thickness, and other measures of obesity in their data collection. In 1960, Stamler and colleagues reported in a study of 784 men employed by a utility corporation that, after 4 years, obese workers had an elevated incidence and prevalence of CHD. Physically active men had slightly lower rates. In the Framingham Study, as summarized by Kannel (1971), cardiovascular disease risk among adults rose progressively with increasing relative weight. Paffenbarger and Wing (1971) have reported that four factors predisposed men to stroke in later life; increased weight for height, cigarette smoking, shorter body structure, and higher levels of blood pressure. The Chicago Stroke Study identified body bulk as a risk factor for stroke (Ostfeld et al., 1974). Stroke risk for these four factors appeared additive. In two reports from the Coronary Drug Project Research Group (1974, 1975), relative body weight did not appear related to mortality or CHD among adult males receiving treatment for previous myocardial infarctions.

Interpretation of data concerning the association between obesity and morbidity and mortality is difficult, however, because obesity is correlated with other risk factors such as blood pressure. Thus it is not entirely clear whether obesity operates directly to cause increased risk, or indirectly through associated factors such as elevated blood pressure level or diabetes.

The Framingham Study (Kannell et al., 1967) suggests that, when unaccompanied by hypertension or hypercholesterolemia, only severe obesity is associated with myocardial infarction. The excess of CHD seen in obese groups in Framingham arose from excess angina pectoris and sudden death. Keys et al. (1972) have noted that obesity made no significant contribution to future CHD when age, blood pressure, serum cholesterol, and smoking were controlled in the International Cooperative Study of Cardiovascular Epidemiology. The Tecumseh study indicated, however, that being overweight increased risk of ischemic heart disease independently of blood pressure, hyperglycemia, or serum cholesterol level (Epstein et al., 1965). The Evans County study (Heyden et al., 1971), in Georgia, shows increased CHD risk among the obese who smoke but not among those who do not smoke.

Whether obesity plays an independent role in stroke seems equally uncertain. Ostfeld (1980) reports that the Framingham cohort shows evidence that obesity contributes to risk of stroke, largely independent of blood pressure. In the Evans County study, on the other hand, much of the association between 20-year weight gain and increased risk of stroke is explained by a concomitant rise in blood pressure (Heyman et al., 1971). In the seven-county survey (Blackburn et al., 1970), obesity was not associated with any form of stroke. However, obesity does seem to aggravate both hypertension and diabetes, both definite risk factors in cardiovascular disease. Thus it plays some role in the development of cardiovascular disease, whether directly or indirectly.

Complicating the interpretation of these findings is the fact that excess weight gain is associated with some diseases (for example, diabetes), whereas low weight or weight loss is associated with other diseases (for example, tuberculosis). Obesity also seems related to social and cultural circumstances. For example, in Tecumseh, well-educated men but less educated women were more obese than other persons of the same sex (Garn et al., 1977). In other studies, however, persons of lower-class showed higher rates of obesity (Khosla and Lowe, 1972; Stunkard et al., 1972). Therefore, associations between obesity and morbidity and mortality may reflect underlying disease or social factors such as lower socioeconomic status.

Alcohol consumption

Alcohol consumption as a factor in people's physical, mental, and social well-being has long aroused concern. In the nineteenth century this concern led to the temperance movement, and ultimately to a trial of prohibition in the United States. Since the turn of the century numerous studies have shown excessive morbidity and mortality associated with heavy alcohol use and alcoholism. The U.S. Department of Health, Education and Welfare, in a recent publication, Alcohol and Health, New Knowledge (1975), reported that consumption of alcohol in large quantities, and alcoholism in particular, are associated with cancer, heart disease, liver and central nervous system disorders, congenital defects, and accidents, as well as with overall mortality. In the last several years some attention has shifted from the effects of heavy consumption to the health effects of more moderate consumption of alcoholic beverages. Much of this research indicates that moderate consumption is not associated with increased disease risk and may, in fact, have some beneficial health effects.

Chronic heavy drinkers, identified on the basis of arrest records, case-finding surveys, clinical situations, or reported drinking habits, have substantially elevated risks of premature death (Schmidt, 1980). For instance, Schmidt and DeLint (1972), comparing deaths of patients after treatment for alcoholism in Toronto with the age-specific mortality rates in the Ontario population as a whole, found that the male mortality ratio was 2.02 times as high as expected; the female ratio was 3.19 times as high. In a prospective study of alcoholism among Dupont Company employees by Pell and D'Alonzo (1973), the mortality ratio among known alcoholics compared to matched controls was 3.61; among suspected alcoholics, 3.10; and among recovered alcoholics, 2.91.

Although studies such as these show an association between alcoholism and mortality, a causal association cannot be inferred with confidence. As Pell and D'Alonzo (1973) state:

Excess morbidity and mortality seen in alcoholics may be due not only to the effects of alcohol itself, but also to certain behavioral and personal characteristics that are more common in alcoholics than nonalcoholics, such as cigarette smoking, use of other drugs, poor dietary habits (leading to nutritional deficiencies), emotional disturbances, and physiological abnormalities that contribute to the development of alcoholism, and concomitantly, to other diseases as well.

In addition, other problems plague studies of alcoholics, the most serious being selection bias (LaPorte et al., 1980). Identification of alcoholics, either in clinical situations or from other sources, often results from the existence of health problems. Alcoholics thus identified are likely to be sicker than those not identified, making any generalizations or causal inferences difficult.

Several prospective population-based studies have indicated a U-shaped relationship between alcohol and mortality, with moderate consumers having the lowest rates. In four groups of adults, two from San Francisco and two nationwide samples, Room and Day (1974) found that both abstainers and frequent, heavy alcohol drinkers experienced higher age and sex-specific mortality rates than did moderate drinkers. The Framingham Study disclosed a weak association between mortality and both abstention and high alcohol use (Kannel, 1971). Other analyses of the Framingham data show that people with alcohol intake greater than

30 ounces per month had significantly fewer myocardial infarctions than those drinking less (Stason et al., 1976).

Several studies of coronary heart disease have yielded either a negative association between that condition and alcohol intake, or again a U-shaped curve. From case-control studies Stason et al. (1976) and Hennekens and co-workers (1978, 1979) report that persons with CHD drank less and had a higher prevalence of abstainers than controls. As other risk factors for the condition are controlled in analyses, a U-shaped curve is obtained, with moderate consumers having the lowest CHD rates. Klatsky and colleagues (1974), using data from a prepaid health plan, also found persons with heart disease more likely to be nondrinkers than controls matched on such demographic factors as age, sex, race, and smoking habits. Yano et al., (1978) have reported a strong negative association between myocardial infarction and alcohol consumption among 7705 Japanese-Americans who are part of the Honolulu Heart Study. The age-adjusted 6-year incidence rates from CHD are greatest for those who consumed little or no alcohol, and they decrease steadily with increasing alcohol consumption. These differences persist when controlling for standard risk factors, including baseline health status.

Marmot and his colleagues (1981) have found that cardiovascular mortality among British civil servants also shows a negative relationship to alcohol consumption. This relationship was independent of age, smoking habit, blood pressure, plasma cholesterol, and grade of employment. However, the increased risk was found only among abstainers. Risk did not decrease further with increasing alcohol consumption. For noncardio-vascular mortality, however, Marmot and co-workers found a strong positive association with alcohol intake. When they examined mortality from all causes in relation to alcohol consumption, a U-shaped curve resulted from the higher cardiovascular mortality in nondrinkers and higher noncardiovascular mortality in heavy drinkers.

Chronic heavy alcohol use has also been reported to be associated with carcinomas, especially of the head, neck, and esophagus (Kissen and Kaley, 1974; Pell and D'Alonzo, 1973; Schmidt and DeLint, 1972). Correlations between these conditions and alcohol use in general populations have also been observed (Lasserre et al., 1967; Schwartz et al., 1966). Most of these studies, however, are subject to the criticism mentioned earlier, namely, the possibility of confounding variables. Wynder and Mabuchi (1972) found no evidence that alcohol alone will increase men's risk of cancer, but they did find that heavy drinking accompanied by smoking significantly increases the risk of cancer of the oral cavity, extrinsic larynx, and esophagus. Other synergistic relationships between smoking and alcohol consumption, and cancer of specific sites have also been reported (Rothman, 1975).

Sleep patterns

Sleep has received relatively little attention as a factor in health and mortality. The two major sources of information on the mortality risk associated with sleeping patterns are the currently described prospective study conducted by the Human Population Laboratory, and a prospective study initiated by the American Cancer Society in 1959–1960, reported by Hammond (1964), Hammond and Garfinkel (1969) and Kripke et al., (1979). In the last and most detailed report of sleeping habits, analyses indicated that men 30 years or older who usually slept less than 4 hours per night were 2.8 times as likely to die within 6 years as those who slept 7 or 8 hours, while those who slept more than 10 hours were 1.8 times as likely to have died. Similar ratios for women were 1.5 and 1.8. These differences remained significant when controlled for age and a history of ever having heart disease, high blood pressure, diabetes, and/or stroke. Analyses also indicated that extremely long or short nightly sleep was associated with mortality from heart disease, stroke, cancer, and suicide.

Studies of sleep deprivation in humans and animals have revealed a decline in temperature and muscular strength, blood chemistry changes, reduced capacity for arousal, and reduced ability to concentrate (Kleitman, 1963). Sleep deprivation ultimately leads to death. It has not always been possible to determine whether the findings are actually due to sleep deprivation or to the means used to keep the person or animal awake—for example, walking on a treadmill. Sleep, though, is clearly necessary for survival.

Hartmann (1973) has summarized several major theories of the function of sleep: (1) to combat fatigue; (2) to form memory, erase excess input, and thereby aid learning; (3) to compensate for energy and oxygen debts; (4) to spread inhibition through the cortex; (5) to allow emergence of repressed unconscious material and biologic needs; and (6) to renew physical and psychological functions. People sleep an average of 7 to 8 hours per night throughout the world, no matter how many hours of daylight are present. Oswald (1976), like Hartmann, believes that slow-wave sleep has a bodily restorative function, whereas rapid-eye-movement (REM or D) sleep is chiefly for brain or psychological repair. Several investigators have found that long sleepers (those who sleep more than 9 hours per night) and short sleepers (who average under 6 hours) have approximately the same number of hours of slow-wave sleep (Baekeland

and Hartmann, 1970, 1971; Hartmann et al., 1971, 1972; Webb and Agnew, 1970). Evidently, long sleepers have more REM sleep. Two studies show that a person's need for sleep increases with stress, depression, or changes in work (Brewer and Hartmann, 1973; Hartmann et al., 1972). The number of hours a person normally sleeps may thus reflect a physical or psychological need. Some individuals deprive themselves of sleep to maintain jobs and activities they desire. Certain illnesses may induce insomnia or excessive sleep, for example, manic-depressive psychosis. Karacan et al., (1976) has shown that trouble with sleeping is more common among those who are black, female, older, in low socioeconomic circumstances, widowed, separated, or divorced.

Eating patterns

Skipping breakfast and other meals regularly has received little attention as a possible factor in determining levels of physical health and mortality risk. Most of the research on eating patterns has been conducted on animals or on small clinic-based populations, with few systematic epidemiologic studies.

Experimental studies reveal that metabolic changes can be induced in different species by altering the frequency of food intake (Cohn and Joseph, 1960; Fabry and Braun, 1967; Leveille, 1972b; Tepperman et al., 1943; Wadhwa et al., 1973). Epidemiologic studies show that large but infrequent meals are associated with overweight (Hejda and Fabry, 1964; Metzner et al., 1977b). In older age groups there is some limited evidence that these same meal patterns are linked to hypercholesterolemia, impaired glucose tolerance, diabetes, increase in serum cholesterol levels, and ischemic heart disease (Fabry and Tepperman, 1970). Studies of young people have suggested that metabolic changes occur in association with changes in feeding frequency (Wadhwa et al., 1973; Young et al., 1972). Nibbling, as opposed to more substantial eating, appeared to be associated with lower serum cholesterol levels. Gorgers exhibited abnormal insulin responses. In other investigations of young obese people, meal frequency did not appear to affect weight loss, nitrogen balance, total serum lipids, or serum cholesterol (Finkelstein and Fryer, 1971; Young et al., 1971a,b). Among young men, a regimen of one meal per day was associated with reduced oral glucose tolerance as well as higher serum cholesterol and serum triglycerides levels, confirming the metabolic studies.

Animal studies indicate that regular meal eating by rats is associated with an increase in body fat, a decrease in body protein and water, and higher levels of serum cholesterol and lipogenic activity (Leveille, 1972a,b).

Meal-fed rats, however, ate less overall than the nibblers, and had lower body weight and increased life span.

In considering studies of eating patterns it should be noted that the normal feeding of most herbivorous animals, including rodents, is nibbling, whereas carnivorous animals typically gorge. Humans are omnivorous animals who apparently started as gorgers during their prehistoric hunting days. Since they began farming, humans evidently have adapted to meal eating.

Health practices and mortality

Introduction

The preceding pages illustrate that a wide range of common habits (practices) are related to health. Although there is considerable and increasing research in this field, several critical issues still need to be examined. These issues involve (1) the influence of health status on behavior; (2) the specificity of disease outcomes associated with health practices; (3) the relationship of health practices with one another, their independence, interactions, and cumulative impact; and (4) social and psychological factors that may influence "risk behaviors." Such questions can be addressed by studying several important health practices simultaneously in one data set—a task we have set for ourselves in this chapter.

It is obvious that many of the health practices may reflect physical health status. For example, illness may cause weight loss, sleep disturbance, and physical inactivity. When diagnosed as having a serious illness, some people change their smoking and drinking habits. Therefore, one must consider the possibility that a certain behavior is related to increased mortality risk only because it is strongly correlated with preexisting illness. In order to examine that hypothesis we have controlled for baseline physical health status in our analyses of individual health practices and subsequent mortality.

A second question is whether health practices affect only specific disease outcomes or have a more general impact on health. Many investigators in this field have assumed either one position or the other, without indicating that the question exists. For example, they study smoking and lung cancer only. Others who assume a general effect examine health practices only in relation to mortality from all causes, or to general levels of physical well-being. Few investigators have dealt directly with the hypothesis that health practices have general disease consequences by examining their impact on mortality from several different causes of death. We will explore this hypothesis by considering separately the risk of dying from four categories of disease: ischemic heart disease, cancer, cerebrovascular and circulatory diseases, and all other causes of death.

A third matter to be examined both in this chapter and in Chapter 5 consists of the interactions of health practices and their independence from one another. Much previous research has focused on only one or two health practices. Rarely have researchers had the opportunity to examine the impact of many behaviors on mortality or morbidity risk. This limitation has meant that we have a very incomplete understanding of their individual contributions. Does physical activity, for instance, have its greatest health effect by reducing weight, as some have thought? In order to direct preventive efforts efficiently, better understanding is needed of the correlations among health practices, their independent contributions, and the way they interact with one another. This major concern we have approached from several directions. In this chapter we will present data on the correlations among seven health practices and the mortality risks associated with each of them individually and in several combinations. In Chapter 5, we will present a multiple logistic risk analysis of these same health practices. In Chapter 6, regression analysis is used to test the hypothesis that health practices predict changes in morbidity as well as differences in mortality.

Fourth is the issue of possible interrelationships between health practices and social and psychological factors in determining health. For example, do people who are alienated or who are poor drink and smoke more, and does the latter relationship account for the association between health practices and mortality? The last part of the chapter deals with that general question, particularly the relationship between groups who maintain high-risk practices and psychological and social variables. The aim is better understanding of the personal characteristics and social conditions associated with the tendency to maintain high-risk behavior.

Another objective was to develop a summary index of significant health practices. There are several reasons for doing this. The first is to facilitate using such an index to describe the overall findings. Another is to measure the cumulative impact of maintaining a number of health practices. Perhaps the most important purpose of a health practices index is to identify groups of people who practice either generally healthy or unhealthy behaviors. Relatively little is known about the personal characteristics or kinds of situations that motivate people to maintain behaviors that, in the long run, will help them to be healthier and live longer. As yet there is little empirical evidence indicating the determinants of "high-risk" or "at risk" behavior. Henderson and Enelow (1976) suggest that cultural and social norms can make such behaviors rewarding, and they can be difficult to change because they are rarely accompanied by the immediate occurrence of serious symptomatology.

As noted in Chapter 2, this monograph focuses on mortality from all causes over a 9-year period as the outcome measure for examining the relationship between health and ways of living. The analysis is further limited to persons who were 30–69 years of age at the time of the survey, 1965. The decision to use that age group arose from several considerations: relatively few deaths occur under age 30; although more than half of all deaths occur at age 70 and beyond, the factors in mortality are even more complex in that period of life than at younger ages; and particular interest in "premature mortality" (death rates up to age 70) has become manifest in the health statistics community.

Obviously the measure of health used, in this case mortality; the period of observation, in this case 1965–1979; and the population examined, in this case a sample of 30- to 69-year-old persons in Alameda County in 1965, may influence what is found about any association that may exist between health and ways of living. For example, Belloc and Breslow (1972) found seven health practices associated with physical health status in the entire Alameda County sample, and Belloc (1973) found these same seven health practices associated with mortality from all causes during the first 5½ years after the 1965 survey. On the other hand, Wiley and Camacho (1980) found five of the same health practices, as determined in 1965, to be significantly associated with physical health status in 1974 among white persons who were under 70 years of age at the time of the 1965 survey.

In this chapter we examine the seven health practices individually in relation to all-cause mortality 1965–1974 in the Alameda County population 30–69 years of age at the time of the 1965 survey. The association between age-adjusted and sex-specific mortality rates will be presented for each health practice, followed by analyses that take into account the 1965 baseline physical health status.

After the health practices have been examined individually, their correlations are presented and their joint contribution to mortality risk is assessed. The health practices that are significantly associated with mortality in this population are combined into an Index of Health Practices. The development and construction of the index is described and age-adjusted mortality rates are presented for men and women. The Health Practices Index is then examined in relation to a series of psychological and social factors, and again in relation to physical health status.

Mortality rates have been age-adjusted by the indirect method suggested by Fleiss (1973) and Lilienfeld (1967) to be most appropriate in analyses that may sometimes involve few cases. Chi-square tests of significance are applied to each of the health practice/mortality analyses. These tests, are based on a Mantel-Haenszel (1959) chi-square statistics, which has been modified by Brand and Sholtz (1976) to adjust for more than two categories of a given variable.

Individual health practices and mortality risk

LEISURE-TIME PHYSICAL ACTIVITY

The 1965 survey included data concerning participation in (1) swimming or walking, (2) physical exercise, (3) sports, (4) gardening, and (5) fishing or hunting. Responses to the items ranged from never to sometimes or often. Swimming or walking, physical exercise, and participation in active sports were weighted equally; gardening and fishing or hunting, because they generally seemed to require substantially less energy expenditure than the others, each received half the weight of the first set of activities. In the Index of Physical Activity a score of 0–3 indicated the least activity; 4–8, moderate activity level; and 9–16, most activity, based on the following:

	Swimming/ walking	Physical	Sports	Gardening	Fishing/ hunting
Never/no answer	0	0	0	0	0
Sometimes	2	2	2	1	1
Often	4	4	4	2	2

It should be noted that only leisure-time activities enter into the index. It thus reflects only a portion of a respondent's total physical activities, excluding activity that is job related and other activities not covered by the survey.

Figure 3-1 reveals a clear gradient of mortality from all causes by extent of activity, for every age and sex group considered. Men aged 30–49 with the lowest level of physical activity experienced 3.1 times the mortality of comparably aged men with the most activity. The relative risk for men 50–59 was 1.9; for men 60–69, 1.7. For women, the relative risks are 3.9 for those aged 30–49, 2.0 for those 50–59, and 2.4 for women 60–69. Thus for both men and women, the relative risks associated with amount of leisure-time physical activity are greatest in the youngest age group and taper off somewhat with increasing age. The difference in age-adjusted mortality

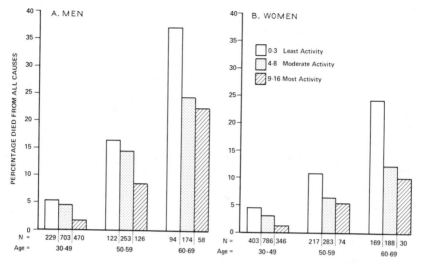

Fig. 3-1. Age- and sex-specific mortality rates from all causes as related to level of leisure-time physical activity: 1965–1974.

between those respondents participating heavily in physical activity and those maintaining low levels of activity was statistically significant for both men and women ($P \leq .005$).

One question, immediately apparent, is whether respondents who did not participate in physical activities were so ill or disabled as to be physically unable to do so. They would thus be more likely to die because their health was already impaired. If this were the case, any association between level of physical activity and mortality that may exist would have little meaning. In order to explore this possibility, the relationship between activity and mortality was examined separately for persons who reported varying degrees of physical health at the time of the 1965 survey. Table 3-1, showing age-adjusted mortality rates from all causes in relation to the Index of Physical Activity and Physical Health Spectrum for both men and women, reveals that the association between physical inactivity and increased mortality risk exists generally among persons in the several categories of the Physical Health Spectrum. Though there is some association between physical inactivity and poor health status, it appears that physical inactivity as measured in the HPL survey is related to mortality independent of physical health status. The relative risk—that is, the gradient of activity with mortality—was greater for those respondents reporting no health problems or only symptoms; it was less with poorer health status, among persons with chronic conditions or disability.

Table 3-1. Age-adjusted mortality rates from all causes (per 100): Level of leisure-time physical activity and Physical Health Spectrum, men and women ages 30–69, 1965–1974

Physical activity level	Disability		Chronic condition		Symptoms only		No health problem		Total	(N)
Men										
Least activity	25.6	(72)	8.5	(155)	9.5	(100)	9.3	(118)	12.4	(445)
Moderate activity	20.3	(63)	7.1	(443)	9.5	(259)	7.5	(365)	9.8	(1130)
Most activity	—	(27)[a]	7.1	(181)	4.9	(186)	3.6	(260)	6.0	(654)
Total (N)	22.8	(162)	8.6	(779)	8.1	(545)	6.5	(743)	9.5	(2229)
Women										
Least activity	15.6	(168)	6.8	(270)	3.8	(200)	8.6	(151)	9.1	(789)
Moderate activity	11.5	(98)	5.0	(465)	5.0	(394)	3.5	(300)	5.3	(1257)
Most activity	—	(26)[a]	6.0	(130)	0.0	(154)	1.9	(140)	3.2	(450)
Total (N)	14.0	(292)	5.8	(865)	3.8	(748)	4.7	(591)	6.4	(2496)

[a]Rates not calculated for cells with 30 or fewer individuals.

CIGARETTE SMOKING

In order to investigate the relationship between smoking and mortality in the Human Population Laboratory sample, respondents were classified according to their smoking history in 1965, that is, past, present, or never; and their risk of dying in the 9-year period following the survey. Amount of cigarettes smoked, years of smoking, and inhalation patterns were also considered.

Figure 3-2 shows age-adjusted, sex-specific mortality rates from all causes according to smoking history. Among both men and women, there is a clear gradient in mortality: present and past smokers experienced generally higher rates than those who had never smoked. The relative risk of mortality among present smokers compared with those who never smoked cigarettes, in the 30–49 age group, was 4.8 for men and 2.9 for women. Among men aged 50–59, the relative risks were lower, 2.3; and among women aged 50–59 past smokers had the highest mortality rates. In the oldest age group, past smokers had mortality rates either about equal to, or greater than, present smokers. Present male smokers had a risk 2.3 times as high as those who never smoked, and female smokers experienced a 1.5 times higher mortality rate than women who had never smoked. The rates also tended to be higher among persons who had quit smoking than among those who had never smoked. The relative risks

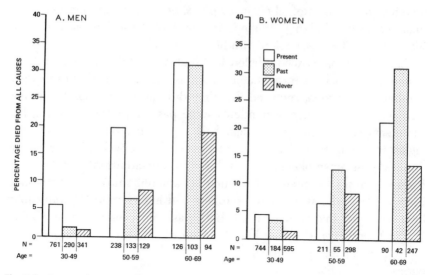

Fig. 3-2. Age- and sex-specific mortality rates from all causes as related to smoking status: 1965–1974.

associated with cigarette smoking were higher for men than women in every age group, and also higher in the younger rather than the older age group ($P \leq .001$ for men and $\leq .01$ for women).

One possible explanation for higher mortality rates among women who were past smokers may have been cessation of smoking because of physical illness. Table 3-2 shows age-adjusted mortality rates according to smoking history and physical health status. Among women in good health —that is, with either no health problems or just symptoms—past smokers had low mortality rates, at least as low as women who had never smoked. Among women reporting chronic conditions or disability, however, past smokers had very high mortality rates. This finding suggests that a substantial proportion of women who quit smoking may have given up the habit because of illness. That could explain the very high mortality rates found among women who are past smokers. Among women in the two healthier categories, however, and among men in all categories on the Physical Health Spectrum, past smokers had mortality rates lower than those of present smokers. These data are consistent with other evidence linking cigarette smoking to poor health. In considering the relationship between cigarette smoking and mortality, it may be useful to examine several characteristics of cigarette smokers other than present smoking status, for example, whether or not respondents inhaled cigarette smoke;

whether they also smoked cigars or pipes; or, perhaps most critical, how many packs per day they smoked. Any or all of these characteristics may play a role in the association with health status.

Cigarette smokers who inhaled had higher mortality rates than those who did not inhale. Approximately twice as high a proportion of women, compared with men, reported that they did not inhale cigarette smoke. This was true whether respondents were past or present smokers. Respondents who smoke more than half a pack per day generally have higher mortality rates than those who smoke half a pack a day or less, or those who never smoke. Table 3-3 shows the age-adjusted mortality rates from all causes for men and women by amount smoked and smoking history. Men who were heavy smokers had higher mortality rates than light smokers; this is evident for both past and present smokers. This gradient, however, does not hold for women.

OBESITY

For testing the hypothesis that people who are obese are at greater risk of dying than persons of average weight, we utilized the Quetelet Index. This measure of obesity adjusts each respondent's weight for height so that people of comparable proportions are coded together. The following quotient, for each respondent, constitutes the Quetelet Index:

$$\left(\frac{\text{Weight in pounds}}{\text{Height in inches}} \right)^2$$

Scores from the Quetelet Index were then arranged in categories, based on Metropolitan Life Insurance reports of desirable mean weights for heights, as follows: (1) 10 percent or more underweight, (2) 9.9 percent underweight to 29.9 percent overweight, and (3) 30.0 percent or more overweight.

Figure 3-3 presents age-specific mortality rates from all causes (per 100) for men and women, according to the Quetelet Index of obesity. People in the average weight-per-height category generally had the lowest mortality rates and the differences among categories were statistically significant for men and women ($P \leq .05$). Respondents in both the underweight and overweight categories experienced an increased risk of dying during the follow-up period, although that higher risk did not extend through all age and sex groups. Among all age and sex groups with the exception of women aged 30–49, underweight respondents were even more likely to die in the follow-up period than were respondents who were obese. However, respondents who were 30 percent overweight were generally more likely to die than respondents who were of moderate weight for height.

Table 3-2. Age-adjusted mortality rates from all causes (per 100): Smoking status and Physical Health Spectrum, men and women ages 30–69, 1965–1974

| | Physical Health Spectrum | | | | | | | | | |
	Disability	(N)	Chronic condition	(N)	Symptoms only	(N)	No health problem	(N)	Total	(N)
Smoking status										
Men										
Present	27.1	(89)	11.1	(376)	11.0	(292)	8.8	(368)	12.8	(1125)
Past	16.2	(35)	7.9	(207)	5.1	(110)	5.4	(174)	7.5	(526)
Never	17.8	(35)	5.6	(191)	4.9	(140)	1.6	(198)	5.5	(564)
Total (N)	22.2	(159)	8.6	(774)	8.1	(542)	6.6	(740)	9.4	(2215)
Women										
Present	14.4	(122)	6.3	(348)	4.0	(342)	8.3	(233)	7.5	(1045)
Past	23.5	(37)	10.2	(97)	3.3	(94)	2.1	(53)	9.5	(281)
Never	11.5	(131)	4.4	(412)	3.5	(306)	2.7	(291)	4.9	(1140)
Total (N)	13.9	(290)	5.8	(857)	3.8	(742)	4.5	(577)	6.4	(2466)

Table 3-3. Age-adjusted mortality rates from all causes (per 100) for men and women ages 30–69: Smoking history and amount smoked (packs/day), men and women ages 30–69, 1965–1974

| | Present | | | | Past | | | | Never | | Total | |
Sex	>½ pack	(N)	<½ pack	(N)	>½ pack	(N)	<½ pack	(N)	0 pack	(N)	Total	(N)
Men	14.5	(836)	8.8	(287)	8.0	(395)	6.5	(125)	5.4	(564)	9.4	(2207)
Women	7.4	(655)	7.6	(385)	10.1	(125)	9.1	(149)	5.0	(1140)	6.3	(2454)

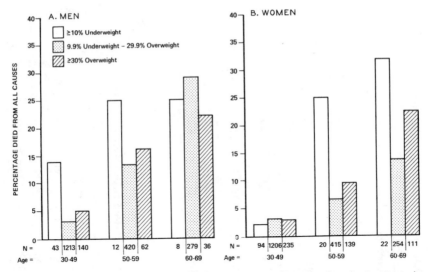

Fig. 3-3. Age- and sex-specific mortality rates from all causes as related to obesity (Quetelet Index): 1965–1974.

A somewhat unexpected finding in this analysis was the relatively high mortality risk associated with being 10 percent or more underweight. In order to ascertain whether this increased risk might be due to poor health status, especially the presence of debilitating disease of respondents who were underweight, the relationship between weight per height and mortality was examined while controlling for health status at the time of the original survey in 1965 (Table 3-4). Unfortunately, there are not enough underweight respondents to analyze their mortality risk within separate categories of the physical health spectrum. However, the numbers within each of the 12 cells in the table indicate a strong association between being underweight and reporting some disability. It appears that respondents who were underweight in 1965 also were in poorer health at that time than their moderate-weight counterparts. Their poor health might thus have been responsible for both being underweight and increased mortality risk.

Also apparent from the mortality rates shown in Table 3-4 is the inconsistent association, especially in men, between obesity and increased mortality risk when controlling for physical health status in 1965. Women in three of the four health status categories who were 30 percent or more overweight had higher mortality rates than respondents in the average-weight-per-height category. Among men, however, the association is not evident in the various health status categories.

Table 3-4. Age-adjusted mortality rates from all causes (per 100): Obesity (Quetelet Index) and Physical Health Spectrum, men and women ages 30–69, 1965–1974

Quetelet Index	Physical Health Spectrum									
	Disability		Chronic condition		Symptoms only		No health problem		Total	(N)
Men										
10% and under	—	(13)[a]	—	(21)[a]	—	(15)[a]	—	(14)[a]	19.1	(63)
Average	22.3	(127)	8.3	(652)	8.0	(469)	6.6	(664)	9.2	(1912)
30% and over	—	(20)[a]	11.4	(102)	7.0	(59)	4.8	(57)	10.0	(238)
Total (N)	22.7	(160)	8.6	(775)	8.2	(543)	6.6	(735)	9.5	(2213)
Women										
10% and under	—	(24)[a]	7.9	(36)	5.6	(38)	0.0	(38)	10.8	(136)
Average	12.9	(174)	5.0	(624)	3.5	(611)	4.9	(466)	5.7	(1875)
30% and over	11.8	(94)	7.6	(205)	4.7	(99)	5.1	(87)	5.7	(485)
Total (N)	14.0	(292)	6.0	(865)	3.8	(748)	4.7	(591)	6.4	(2496)

[a]Rates not calculated for cells with 30 or fewer individuals.

ALCOHOL CONSUMPTION

In order to assess the association between alcohol consumption and mortality risk in the HPL survey population, a measure of alcohol intake was constructed using several questions concerning both frequency and quantity of liquor, wine, and beer consumption. This measure differs somewhat from the measure of alcohol consumption used in previous HPL publications concerning physical health status in 1965 and mortality follow-up.

For purposes of this present analysis, alcohol consumption was determined by responses to two sets of questions: (1) "How often do you drink wine, beer, or liquor?" and (2) "When you drink wine, beer, or liquor, how many drinks do you usually have at a sitting?" An index of alcohol consumption was created by summing up the volume of beer, wine, and liquor usually drunk by an individual. This volume for each type of alcohol was computed by multiplying the frequency by the average volume, with frequency and volume coded as follows:

Frequency		Volume	
Never	0.0	Never	0.0
Less than once per week	2.5	One or two drinks	1.5
Once or twice per week	7.0	Three or four drinks	3.5
More than twice per week	15.0	Five plus drinks	6.0

The index for an individual could hence range from 0 to 270, with a score of 0 to 90 for each of the three types of alcohol consumed.

This index, based on measures of both frequency and quantity of alcohol ingestion as well as cut-off points in the formation of categories, generally follows the results of studies of drinking practices conducted by Cahalan and Cisin (1968). The omission of "highest amount drunk" is the major departure in the HPL index of alcohol consumption from the index developed by Cahalan and Cisin. For most analyses reported here the responses were divided into three categories: (1) those abstaining from alcohol consumption or with a drinking index of 16 or less; (2) those with a drinking index between 17 and 45; and (3) those whose index was 46 or more.

Age- and sex-specific mortality rates for each level of alcohol consumption appear in Figure 3-4. For most age and sex categories, moderate drinkers had the lowest mortality rates. With the exception of women aged 50-59, persons who never drank alcoholic beverages or who drank lightly had mortality rates somewhat higher than moderate drinkers. The highest mortality rates occurred among respondents whose drinking index exceeded 46. The mortality risk associated with heavy drinking of alcoholic beverages was especially high among men in the age group 30-49, almost five times as high as that of moderate drinkers. The relative risks associated with alcohol consumption were generally greater for men than for women. When adjusted for age, the mortality rate among men who drank moderately was clearly lower than the mortality rate of the two other groups of men, abstainers and light drinkers, or heavier drinkers ($P \leq .001$), but uncertainly so in the case of women ($P \leq .05$).

Persons with an index of 60 or more had even higher mortality rates than those whose index was between 46 and 60 (Table 3-5). Again, it is apparent that the relative risk associated with very heavy drinking is greater for men than for women.

Abstainers and light drinkers conceivably could have had higher mortality rates than moderate drinkers because of health conditions for which they were advised to abstain from alcoholic beverages, or possibly their physical conditions caused them to change their drinking habits. Age-adjusted mortality from all causes was therefore examined in relation to the index of alcohol consumption among persons on various segments of the Physical Health Spectrum, the HPL measure of physical health status (Table 3-6). Among men in every category of health status, abstainers and light drinkers had higher mortality rates than moderate drinkers. Thus it does not appear that the increased mortality rate among men who either abstained totally from alcohol beverage consumption or drank very lightly was the result of poor physical health status in 1965. Among

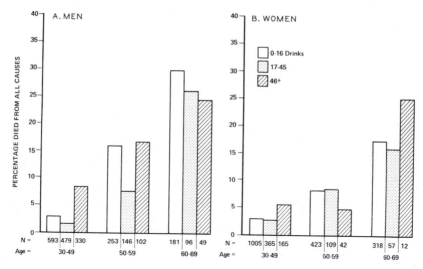

Fig. 3-4. Age- and sex-specific mortality rates from all causes as related to alcohol consumption. 1965–1974.

women, abstainers and light drinkers died at a rate similar to that of moderate drinkers.

SLEEPING PATTERN

Not much attention has been given to sleep pattern as a possible factor in health. Poor sleep often seems to result from poor health, to be a symptom rather than a cause of illness.

The HPL questionnaire included the following question: "How many hours of sleep do you usually get at night?" with responses coded into four categories: (1) 6 hours or less, (2) 7 hours, (3) 8 hours, (4) 9 hours or more. For purposes of analysis, those sleeping 7 or 8 hours a night comprised one category; and those sleeping less or more, the other two.

Age-specific mortality rates for men and women according to hours of sleep per night appear in Figure 3-5. Both men and women who reported

Table 3-5. Age-adjusted mortality rates from all causes (per 100): Alcohol consumption, men and women, ages 30–69, 1965–1974

Sex	Drinking index							
	0–16	(N)	17–45	(N)	46–60	(N)	61–270	(N)
Men	9.9	(1027)	6.6	(721)	8.3	(167)	14.9	(337)
Women	6.4	(1746)	6.1	(531)	6.0	(531)	10.4	(129)

Table 3-6. Age-adjusted mortality rates from all causes (per 100): Alcohol consumption index and Physical Health Spectrum, men and women ages 30–69, 1965–1974

Drinking index	Physical Health Spectrum									
	Disability		Chronic condition		Symptoms		No health problem		Total	(N)
Men										
0–16	21.1	(95)	10.2	(355)	7.1	(232)	6.2	(345)	9.9	(1027)
17–45	17.5	(36)	6.0	(260)	6.8	(180)	4.1	(245)	6.6	(721)
46 +	35.6	(31)	9.7	(164)	12.0	(133)	11.9	(153)	13.3	(481)
Total (N)	22.8	(162)	8.6	(779)	8.2	(545)	6.5	(743)	9.5	(2229)
Women										
0–16	13.0	(232)	5.6	(610)	4.2	(480)	4.3	(424)	6.4	(1746)
17–45	11.9	(42)	6.3	(185)	2.6	(183)	5.7	(121)	6.0	(531)
46 +	—	(18)[a]	5.4	(70)	3.6	(85)	6.4	(46)	8.5	(219)
Total (N)	14.0	(292)	5.8	(865)	3.8	(748)	4.8	(591)	6.4	(2496)

[a]Rates not calculated for cells with 30 or fewer individuals.

that they usually slept 7 or 8 hours each night had significantly lower mortality rates than either respondents reporting 6 or less hours of sleep, or those with 9 or more hours of sleep per night ($P \leq .01$). The only exception to this pattern was among women aged 30–49 who reported 7 or 8 hours of sleep; their mortality rate was essentially the same as the rate for persons reporting 9 or more hours of sleep per night. Persons reporting 6 or less hours of sleep per night experienced generally the highest mortality rates, with the excess being most pronounced in the youngest age group.

Individuals reporting either 6 or less, or 9 or more hours of sleep per night, of course, might have had higher mortality because their physical health status was generally poor in 1965. To explore that hypothesis, age-adjusted mortality rates from all causes for men and women were obtained according to sleeping practices and physical health status in 1965. The results appear in Table 3-7. Without exception, in every category of physical health status, those with 6 or less hours of sleep per night experienced higher mortality rates than those with 7 or 8 hours. With only two exceptions, persons who said they slept 9 or more hours per night also experienced higher mortality than those who reported 7 to 8 hours of sleep. Thus the association between 6 or less, or 9 or more, hours of sleep per night and increased mortality does not appear to be due to differences in physical health status in 1965.

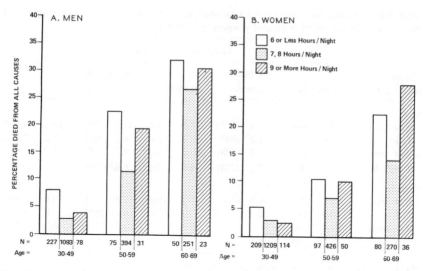

Fig. 3-5. Age- and sex-specific mortality rates from all causes as related to sleeping (hours per night): 1965–1974.

EATING REGULARLY: BREAKFAST AND SNACKING

Eating regular meals, including breakfast, and not snacking between meals has long been part of American folk wisdom. Evidence indicating the relationship of these habits to health status, however, has been minimal. To test whether eating breakfast and eating regularly might contribute to good physical health, two items were included in the 1965 HPL question-naire: (1) "How often do you eat breakfast?" and (2) "How often do you eat in between your regular meals?" Responses to each of these items were then scored as (1) "almost every day," (2) "sometimes" or "once in a while," and (3) "rarely or never." In reports of previous analyses of HPL data, based on a sample of the entire population of Alameda County over 20 years of age, these two variables were shown to be associated both with physical health status in 1965 and with mortality during the first 5½ years of follow-up (Belloc, 1973; Belloc and Breslow, 1972). Individuals who generally ate breakfast and did not snack between meals reported better physical health and experienced lower mortality than did persons with less regular eating habits.

In order to examine the relationship of these items to mortality during the 9-year follow-up period (1965–1974) among persons 30–69 years of age, age-specific mortality rates from all causes were tabulated for both men and women with respect to each of the two health practices. Figure 3-6 shows that in general those who reported eating breakfast almost daily

Table 3-7. Age-adjusted rates from all causes (per 100): Sleeping (hours per night) and Physical Health Spectrum, men and women ages 30–69, 1965–1974

Sleeping (hrs/night)	Physical Health Spectrum										
	Disability		Chronic condition		Symptoms		No health problem		Total	(N)
Men										
6 or less	24.9	(44)	13.4	(137)	11.1	(88)	11.1	(83)	14.8	(352)
7–8	21.0	(100)	7.9	(592)	6.7	(423)	6.1	(623)	8.2	(1738)
9 or more	—	(18)[a]	3.5	(45)	15.2	(34)	6.7	(35)	11.2	(132)
Total (N)	22.6	(162)	10.2	(774)	8.0	(545)	6.6	(741)	9.4	(2222)
Women										
6 or less	14.7	(80)	6.9	(162)	5.3	(101)	7.5	(43)	9.0	(386)
7–8	12.0	(178)	5.4	(630)	3.9	(598)	4.1	(499)	5.6	(1905)
9 or more	21.4	(32)	6.5	(72)	0.0	(49)	7.4	(47)	8.5	(200)
Total (N)	13.8	(290)	5.8	(864)	3.8	(748)	4.7	(589)	6.4	(2491)

[a]Rates not calculated for cells with 30 or fewer individuals.

had lower mortality rates than the others who ate breakfast only sometimes, rarely, or never. With the exception of men in the category 50–59 years old, however, individuals who sometimes ate breakfast appeared to have mortality rates slightly higher than those who ate breakfast either regularly or never. This finding suggests that it may not be eating breakfast per se that is associated with mortality, but rather the regularity with which one does or does not eat breakfast. The differences in mortality rates among the three groups were not substantial and reached a probability of .07 for men and .22 for women, compared with the standard of statistical significance, $P \leq .05$.

Examination of the relationship between eating breakfast and mortality while controlling for physical health status in 1965 does not seem to affect the finding (Table 3-8). Within each category of physical health, those respondents who reported that they almost always ate breakfast experienced generally lower mortality rates.

Age-specific mortality rates from all causes according to the extent of snacking appear in Figure 3-7. There appears to be no consistent relationship between frequency of snacking between meals and mortality. The difference in mortality rates among the three groups was not statistically significant $(P \geq .05)$.

In order to examine whether the previously reported association between snacking and mortality might be in some way hidden because of some relationship between physical health status, snacking, and mortality, the possible association was reassessed while controlling for physical

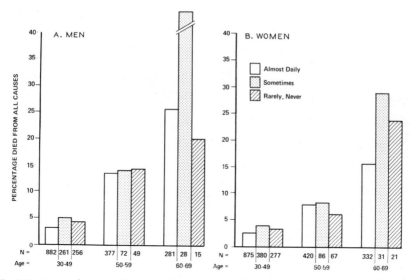

Fig. 3-6. Age- and sex-specific mortality rates from all causes as related to eating breakfast: 1965–1974.

Table 3-8. Age-adjusted mortality rates from all causes (per 100): Eating breakfast and Physical Health Spectrum, men and women ages 30–69, 1965–1974

Eating break-fast frequency	Physical Health Spectrum									
	Disability		Chronic condition		Symptoms		No health problem		Total	(N)
Men										
Almost always	20.9	(114)	8.2	(565)	7.1	(347)	6.0	(514)	8.7	(1540)
Sometimes	45.1	(33)	10.9	(119)	10.5	(96)	7.1	(113)	12.8	(361)
Rarely or never	—	(14)ᵃ	8.5	(93)	10.4	(100)	8.2	(113)	9.9	(320)
Total (N)	22.8	(161)	8.6	(777)	8.3	(543)	6.4	(740)	9.4	(2221)
Women										
Almost always	14.2	(196)	5.0	(576)	4.4	(457)	3.9	(398)	5.9	(1627)
Sometimes	7.6	(48)	12.7	(174)	3.2	(158)	6.2	(117)	8.1	(497)
Rarely or never	16.9	(46)	6.0	(114)	1.4	(130)	5.9	(75)	6.4	(365)
Total (N)	13.7	(290)	5.7	(864)	3.8	(745)	4.4	(590)	6.3	(2489)

ᵃRates are not calculated for cells with 30 or fewer individuals.

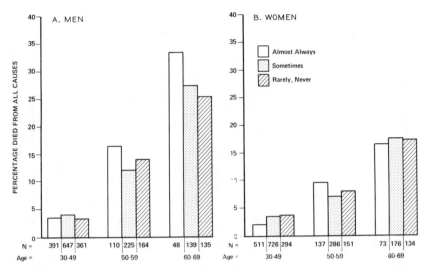

Fig. 3-7. Age- and sex-specific mortality rates from all causes as related to snacking: 1965–1974.

health status in 1965. Table 3-9 does not show any association between snacking and mortality risk while controlling for original level of physical health status.

The data concerning the relationship between snacking and eating breakfast and the risk of mortality among persons 30–69 years of age during the 1965–1974 follow-up period suggest that eating habits, measured in the limited manner of the 1965 HPL survey, do not carry as important a mortality risk in the age group studied as the other five health practices. For neither of the two habits were the chi-square values pertaining to differences in mortality statistically significant. Furthermore, the patterns in mortality risk among the response categories were inconsistent. In comparison with the other five health practices that were examined, eating breakfast and snacking between meals did not appear as strongly associated with risk of dying over the follow-up period. It should be noted, however, that the two questionnaire items used may not have been very good measures of eating patterns. Clearly, they do not measure the adequacy of an individual's diet. From the limited findings reported here it appears that the matter of regularity in eating, whether this includes breakfast and snacking or not, deserves further study.

Thus, of the seven health practices examined in this chapter, five were strongly and with statistical significance associated with mortality from all causes. In no case did a significant association between mortality and each

Table 3-9. Age-adjusted mortality rates from all causes (per 100): Snacking and Physical Health Spectrum, men and women ages 30–69, 1965–1974

Snacking frequency	Physical Health Spectrum									
	Disability		Chronic condition		Symptoms		No health problem		Total	(N)
Men										
Almost daily	26.9	(42)	9.2	(188)	7.8	(168)	7.8	(151)	10.6	(549)
Sometimes	23.4	(69)	8.5	(352)	6.8	(230)	7.6	(360)	9.2	(1011)
Rarely or never	20.1	(50)	8.6	(236)	8.3	(145)	3.8	(229)	8.9	(660)
Total (N)	23.1	(161)	8.6	(776)	8.3	(543)	6.4	(740)	9.4	(2220)
Women										
Almost daily	15.7	(74)	4.4	(234)	3.2	(260)	4.9	(153)	5.9	(721)
Sometimes	11.8	(127)	7.3	(420)	4.7	(346)	3.6	(295)	6.5	(1188)
Rarely or never	15.4	(88)	4.2	(210)	2.8	(139)	6.0	(142)	6.7	(579)
Total (N)	14.0	(289)	5.8	(864)	3.8	(745)	4.7	(590)	6.4	(2488)

of the health practices seem wholly the result of poor health status at the time of the 1965 survey, although it appeared that in some cases poor physical health status might have influenced certain of the practices.

The cumulative impact of health practices

The analyses reported in the preceding section prompted further investigation of the health practices and their relationship to mortality. Of particular interest was the interrelationship of the health practices, their independence from one another, and the cumulative effects they may have on mortality risk. It also seemed desirable to have a summary measure of the health practices, which then could be used for several purposes, ranging from general assessment of health risks to examining the association between overall "health behavior" and other social and psychological factors.

As already noted, five of the seven practices were significantly associated with mortality in the age group 30–69 over the 9 years of the study, in most cases for both men and women. Furthermore, the relationship between each health practice and mortality remained substantially unaffected when physical health status at the time of the survey was controlled. The five health practices were (1) physical activity, (2) cigarette smoking, (3) alcohol consumption, (4) weight/height, and (5) sleeping patterns.

An important question not yet considered is whether some underlying connection among the health practices themselves could be causing spurious associations between any of the individual health practices and mortality. For example, the relationship of excessive drinking with mortality might merely reflect the association of such drinking with cigarette smoking. To investigate that kind of issue another set of analyses was required.

The first step was simply to determine which, if any, of the practices were highly correlated with one another. Table 3-10 shows Pearson product-moment partial correlations for each of the seven health practices with one another, while controlling for age. These correlations are generally small, indicating weak relationships among the health practices. The only items showing moderate correlations are smoking, drinking, and not eating breakfast. To some extent people who smoke cigarettes also tend to drink heavily and skip breakfast.

The relationship between each of the health practices and mortality was then examined while holding constant the six other health practices. Although the data are too extensive to be complete here, the results indicate that each of the five health practices was associated with mortality independently of the other health practices. (That was not true of eating breakfast and snacking.) For example, Table 3-11 shows the relationship of physical activity to mortality while controlling for the other six health practices. Thus the five health practices appeared to make independent contributions to the risk of dying among persons 30–69 years of age over the period between 1965 and 1974.

CONSTRUCTION OF A HEALTH PRACTICES INDEX

In order to simplify the construction of a Health Practices Index, each of the five health practices found to be strong, independent predictors of mortality was recoded as a dichotomous variable and then scored as 0 or 1. Every respondent received a health practices score based on the number of low-risk health practices reported. Although it was evident that the health practices did not each make an equal contribution to the mortality risk, in this index each habit was weighted equally.

Table 3-12 shows the five health practices lined up as dichotomous variables, and the age-adjusted mortality rates among men and women for each of the newly coded health practices. Persons in the sample were coded into two groups with respect to cigarette smoking: (1) those who smoked (including past and present), and (2) those who had never smoked cigarettes. The weight-for-height item groups those respondents who are either overweight or underweight, and those of average weight. Alcohol consumption was recorded so that abstainers, light and moderate drinkers

Table 3-10. Correlations among health practices (controlling for age) for men and women ages 30–69, 1965

High-risk practices	Smokes cigarettes	Overweight	Drinking index 46 +	Physically inactive	Sleeps ≥ 9 or ≤ 6 hrs/night	Skips breakfast	Snacks frequently
Men							
Smokes cigarettes	1.00						
Overweight	-.07	1.00					
Drinking index 46 +	.14	.01	1.00				
Physically inactive	-.09	-.03	-.04	1.00			
Sleeps ≥ 9 or ≤ 6 hrs/night	-.07	.00	-.03	-.03	1.00		
Skips breakfast	.20	.07	.11	.07	-.10	1.00	
Snacks frequently	-.03	.04	-.07	.01	-.05	.00	1.00
Women							
Smokes cigarettes	1.00						
Overweight	-.08	1.00					
Drinking index 46 +	.22	-.09	1.00				
Physically inactive	-.01	.07	-.08	1.00			
Sleeps ≥ 9 or ≤ 6 hrs/night	-.02	.03	.03	-.04	1.00		
Skips breakfast	.22	.03	.08	.07	-.10	1.00	
Snacks frequently	-.06	.01	-.08	-.04	.01	-.04	1.00

Table 3-11. Age-adjusted mortality rates from all causes (per 100): Number of health practices and physical activity level, men and women ages 30–69, 1965–1974

Number of low-risk health practices	Physical activity level							
	Least activity	(0–3)	Moderate activity	(4–8)	Most activity	(9–16)	Total (N)	
Men								
0–3	17.01	(205)	12.4	(486)	7.5	(241)	12.5	(932)
4	16.5	(148)	9.8	(380)	7.1	(224)	8.8	(752)
5, 6	10.8	(92)	6.3	(264)	3.4	(189)	6.5	(545)
Total (N)	12.4	(445)	9.8	(1130)	6.0	(654)	9.5	(2229)
Women								
0–3	11.4	(351)	7.0	(470)	6.5	(165)	9.6	(986)
4	8.4	(245)	4.8	(407)	1.2	(147)	5.5	(799)
5, 6	6.6	(193)	4.5	(380)	2.5	(138)	4.9	(711)
Total (N)	9.1	(789)	5.2	(1257)	3.2	(450)	6.4	(2496)

(i.e., those with drinking index between 0 and 45) were in one category; those whose Drinking Index was 46 or more formed the other group. On the physical activity measure, persons who scored from 5 to 16 were placed in the high-activity category; and those with 0–4, in light activity. Finally, those who slept 7 or 8 hours per night constituted one category, and those who reported obtaining less than 7, or more than 9 hours of sleep the other.

Each low-risk health behavior counted as one point. Thus a point was given for never smoking, being of average weight per height, Drinking Index 0–45, scoring 5–16 on the Index of Physical Activity, and sleeping 7 or 8 hours per night.

As shown in Figure 3-8, there are no major age or sex differences in the Index of Health Practices. Examination of individual health practices, however, does indicate some sex differences in the percentage of people engaging in certain health practices. For example, women are more likely than men to be overweight but less likely either to smoke cigarettes or to drink heavily.

Figure 3-9 portrays age- and sex-specific mortality from all causes according to the Index of Health Practices, that is, among persons who reported (a) 0, 1, or 2 low-risk health practices, (b) 3 low-risk health practices, and (c) 4 or 5 low-risk health practices. There was a strong and consistently lower mortality with increasing number of low-risk health practices. The risk of mortality among men 30–49 years of age with only 0–2 low-risk health practices was 8.4 times as high as that among men of the same age who reported 4–5; for men aged 50–59 and 60–69 the relative

Table 3-12. Age-adjusted mortality rates from all causes (per 100) for each health practice used in Index of Health Practices, men and women ages 30–69, 1965–1974

Health practice	Men	(N)	Women	(N)
Smoking cigarettes				
Never	5.5	(564)	4.9	(1140)
Ever	10.9	(1651)	7.9	(1326)
Weight/height				
Average	9.2	(1912)	5.7	(1875)
Over/under	11.6	(301)	8.3	(621)
Alcohol consumption				
0–45	8.6	(1748)	6.3	(2277)
46 +	13.2	(301)	8.3	(621)
Physical activity				
5–16 High	8.0	(1568)	3.9	(1399)
0–4 Low	12.0	(661)	8.6	(1097)
Sleeping				
7, 8 hrs/night	8.2	(1738)	5.5	(1905)
More, less	13.6	(434)	8.8	(586)

risks were 2.4 and 1.7, respectively. For women, the corresponding relative risks were 2.9, 2.0, and 4.0. Adjusted for age, the chi square for the differences in mortality rates among those with varying health practice scores was highly significant for both men and women ($P \leq .001$).

These findings substantiate a strong relationship between health practices and mortality risk. Although the Index of Health Practices is not identical to that used in previous HPL reports, the present findings are very similar to those previously reported. In the following pages, several other factors will be examined in order to assess whether the powerful association between health practices and mortality might be due to certain confounding variables.

The meaning of the association between health practices and mortality

The explanation for the association between health practices and mortality is by no means self-evident. Following low-risk health practices may favorably influence health. Another hypothesis that comes immediately to mind, however, is that people with poor health practices follow them because of their poor physical health status. For example, people who are physically inactive or underweight may be sick and thus unable to be more active or maintain normal weight. This hypothesis concerning the direction of influ-

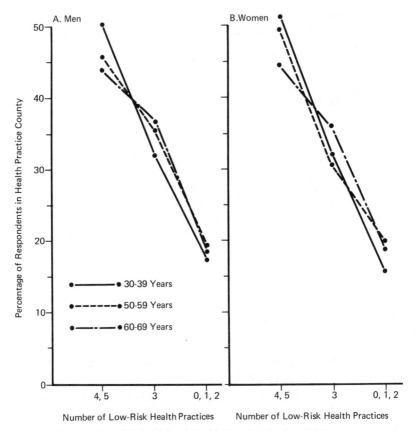

Fig. 3-8. Age and sex distribution of Health Practices Index: 1965.

ence in the association is difficult to assess, but two further analyses throw some light on the relationship between health practices and mortality.

First, the relationship between the Health Practices Index and mortality was examined while controlling for physical health status at the time of the survey in 1965. The latter was assessed by the Physical Health Spectrum, an index developed as a measure of general physical health.

Age-adjusted mortality rates from all causes appear in Table 3-13, separately for each category of the Health Practices Index and Physical Health Spectrum. In every level of health status, both men and women with the most low-risk health practices had lower mortality rates than those with high-risk health practices. Furthermore, the gradient from high to low is consistent through 23 of the 24 cells representing the four degrees of health status and the three health practice categories. It is statistically highly significant ($P \leq .001$). Thus the association between health practice

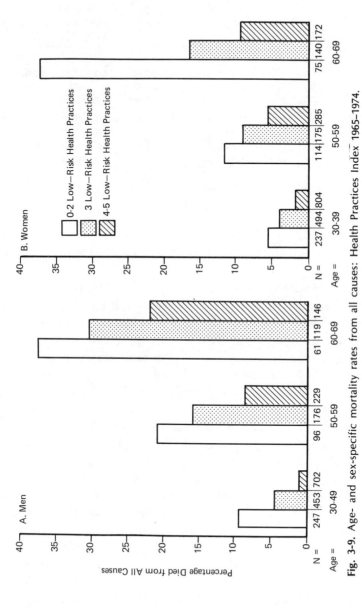

Fig. 3-9. Age- and sex-specific mortality rates from all causes: Health Practices Index 1965–1974.

Table 3-13. Age-adjusted mortality rates from all causes (per 100): Health Practices Index and Physical Health Spectrum, men and women ages 30–69, 1965–1974

Number of low-risk health practices	Physical Health Spectrum									
	Disability		Chronic condition		Symptoms		No health problems		Total	
	%	(N)	%	(N)	%	(N)	%	(N)	%	(N)
Men										
0, 1, 2	28.5	(58)	10.4	(157)	15.5	(91)	16.3	(98)	16.0	(404)
3	24.1	(56)	10.3	(264)	7.8	(200)	8.4	(228)	10.9	(748)
4, 5	13.8	(48)	6.6	(358)	5.7	(254)	3.4	(417)	5.8	(1077)
Total (N)	22.8	(162)	8.7	(779)	8.1	(545)	6.5	(743)	9.5	(2229)
Women										
0, 1, 2	18.5	(100)	10.0	(157)	5.5	(105)	8.0	(64)	11.9	(426)
3	15.0	(105)	5.7	(296)	2.8	(233)	7.9	(175)	7.1	(809)
4, 5	5.7	(87)	4.3	(412)	3.9	(410)	2.6	(352)	3.9	(1261)
Total (N)	14.0	(292)	5.7	(865)	3.8	(748)	4.7	(591)	6.4	(2496)

score and mortality in the subsequent 9½ years holds irrespective of original physical health status.

A second approach to this problem was to examine health practices and mortality according to year of death. If severe physical illness (and therefore likelihood of dying) in 1965 were responsible for poor health practices at the time of the baseline survey, it would reasonably be expected that people in such poor health (and thus with poor health practices) would die mostly in the early years following the survey. Table 3-14 does not bear that out. Of the persons who died during the follow-up period and who reported high-risk health practices, only a relatively small proportion of them died during the earliest years following the survey. Most deaths among those with high-risk health practices occurred in the later years. Though not conclusive, these findings suggest that physical illness at the time of the survey does not account for the association between the habits and mortality. The figures in this table are not adjusted for age; however, it has previously been shown that the Health Practices Index is associated with mortality independently of age. Furthermore, earlier analyses of the data throughout the 9-year follow-up period, including the final 4-year period (Breslow and Enstrom, 1980), revealed the persistence of mortality association.

Another important question about the association is whether it holds for death generally, or can be accounted for by one or two causes of death. For example, ischemic heart disease caused about 30 percent of all deaths during the period of study. Association of health practices with mortality as a whole might actually be due to one or two such disease-specific

Table 3-14. Distribution of Health Practices Index responses: Year of death for men and women, ages 30–69, 1965–1974

Number of low-risk health practices	Year of death										Total deaths	
	1965–1966		1967–1968		1969–1970		1971–1972		1973–1974			
	%	(N)	%	(N)	%	(N)	%	(N)	%	(N)	%	(N)
Men												
0, 1, 2	19	(13)	21	(14)	22	(15)	24	(16)	12	(8)	100	(66)
3	17	(15)	16	(14)	18	(16)	32	(28)	14	(12)	100	(85)
4, 5	11	(7)	21	(13)	18	(11)	16	(10)	31	(19)	100	(60)
Women												
0, 1, 2	12	(7)	16	(9)	24	(14)	22	(12)	25	(12)	100	(54)
3	10	(6)	15	(9)	23	(14)	25	(15)	25	(15)	100	(59)
4, 5	10	(5)	25	(12)	21	(10)	19	(9)	23	(11)	100	(47)

associations. In order to resolve this question, age-adjusted mortality rates for four group-causes of death (ischemic heart disease, other circulatory diseases, cancer, and all other causes of death) were computed for persons who followed health practices to varying extents. Table 3-15 reveals for each of the four group-causes of death a consistent and substantial gradient in mortality, ranging from high mortality rates for persons with high-risk health practices, to moderate rates among those with intermediate health practices, and to low death rates among those with low-risk health prac-

Table 3-15. Age-adjusted cause-specific mortality rates (per 100): Number of low-risk health practices, men and women ages 30–69, 1965–1974

Number of low-risk health practices	Cause of death					
	Ischemic heart disease	Cerebrovascular, circulatory	Cancer	Other[a]	Total	(N)
Men						
0, 1, 2	5.2	2.2	2.6	5.7	16.0	(404)
3	4.4	1.5	1.9	3.1	10.9	(748)
4, 5	2.2	0.5	1.5	1.6	5.8	(1077)
Total	3.6	1.1	1.8	2.9	9.5	(2229)
Women						
0, 1, 2	4.2	1.4	2.6	3.8	11.9	(426)
3	1.4	1.1	2.0	2.6	7.1	(809)
4, 5	0.7	0.6	1.4	1.1	3.9	(1261)
Total	1.6	1.0	1.8	2.1	6.4	(2496)

[a]Other causes of death include diseases of respiratory and digestive systems, accidents, suicide.

tices. Thus it appears that the health practice score is predictive of mortality from a wide range of diseases, not just one or two.

These findings support the idea that the association between high-risk health practices and increased mortality rates is not attributable simply to being sick at the time of initial survey, and therefore unable to practice better health habits and destined to die soon. Furthermore, the data shown in Table 3-15 suggest that high-risk health practices have fatal consequences from a wide range of conditions.

RELATIONSHIP BETWEEN HEALTH PRACTICES
AND SOCIAL CLASS AND RACE

The extent to which a person maintains certain health habits may reflect his or her social class and ethnic group. Such underlying factors could possibly be responsible for the association with health status. People in the lowest socioeconomic level have generally higher mortality rates than the rest of the population. Blacks and other minority groups also have higher mortality as a whole. In order to discern the interrelationships among these variables, the association between health practices and mortality was examined while holding constant socioeconomic status and race.

Measures of income and educational level provided an index of socioeconomic status. Each of the measures—that is, income and educational level—were divided into five categories approximating a normal curve so that the middle category contained approximately a third of the sample, the two surrounding groups each included about 20 percent, and the two extreme categories the remainder. An index of socioeconomic status with five categories was then constructed by combining the measures of income and education.

The interrelationships of socioeconomic status, health practices, and mortality are shown here in Figure 3-10 and Table 3-16. Generally, the lower the socioeconomic level the more likely is a person to have high-risk health practices, that is, to score 0–2 on the Index of Health Practices. This relationship is strongest among young people: those in the lowest socioeconomic class are 3–4 times as likely as those in the highest socioeconomic class to report high-risk health practices. In the older age groups the gradient tapers off.

As shown in Table 3-16, however, within each socioeconomic category persons who reported few (0–2) low-risk health practices had higher mortality rates than those who reported 4–5 such health practices. In general, the middle groups (those reporting 3 low-risk health practices) had a mortality rate falling between the high and low health practice groups. After adjusting for both age and socioeconomic status, the differences in these rates are statistically significant both for men and women

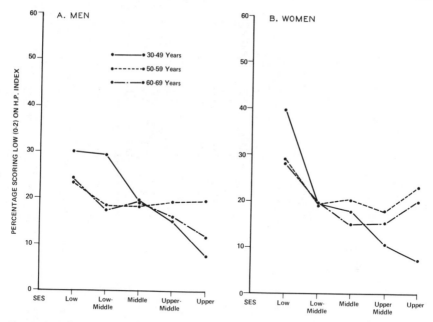

Fig. 3-10. Relationship between Health Practices Index and socioeconomic status (SES) by age and sex: 1965.

($P \leq .001$). Thus the health practice score predicts mortality independently of socioeconomic level.

Table 3-17 shows the age-adjusted mortality rates for each level of the Health Practices Index by race. Again, the mortality/health practice gradient can be seen clearly within most ethnic groups. It is weakest for black women, and not evident among women with racial identity other than black or white. Whereas the table shows that black men and women are much more likely to engage in high-risk health practices than other groups, health practices are associated with mortality independently of race.

HEALTH PRACTICES AND USE
OF PREVENTIVE HEALTH SERVICES

The relationship between health practices and mortality could possibly also be due to failure to use certain medical services by people who maintain high-risk health habits. In order to test this hypothesis, two questions concerning the use of preventive health services were formed into an index (described in greater detail in Chapter 2) indicating the pattern of such services used by respondents. The two questions were as follows: "When was the last time you went to a dentist just for a general

Table 3-16. Age-adjusted mortality rates from all causes (per 100): Health Practices Index and socioeconomic status, men and women ages 30–69, 1965–1974

Number of low-risk health practices	Socioeconomic status											
	Lower	(N)	Low-middle	(N)	Middle	(N)	Upper-middle	(N)	Upper	(N)	Total	(N)
Men												
0, 1, 2	14.3	(45)	14.5	(65)	20.8	(142)	10.0	(117)	—	(24)[a]	15.7	(393)
3	10.4	(77)	16.5	(90)	8.4	(256)	14.0	(241)	2.3	(72)	11.0	(736)
4, 5	5.4	(53)	7.5	(123)	5.7	(346)	5.7	(382)	3.8	(163)	5.7	(1067)
Total (N)	9.9	(175)	11.7	(278)	9.5	(744)	9.1	(740)	5.2	(259)	9.4	(2196)
Women												
0, 1, 2	17.8	(59)	8.7	(69)	12.7	(162)	7.2	(100)	—	(19)[a]	11.5	(409)
3	5.3	(64)	6.5	(128)	7.6	(315)	5.7	(247)	9.1	(41)	6.7	(795)
4, 5	5.4	(67)	1.5	(163)	3.5	(441)	4.3	(469)	3.2	(103)	3.6	(1243)
Total (N)	8.8	(190)	4.6	(360)	6.8	(918)	5.2	(816)	5.3	(163)	6.1	(2447)

[a]Rates not calculated for cells with 30 or fewer individuals.

Table 3-17. Age-adjusted mortality rates from all causes (per 100): Health Practices Index and race, men and women ages 30–69, 1965–1974

Number of low-risk health practices	Race							
	White	(N)	Black	(N)	Other	(N)	Total	(N)
Men								
0, 1, 2	15.9	(307)	19.4	(73)	—	(24)[a]	16.0	(404)
3	10.7	(580)	10.0	(110)	15.3	(58)	10.9	(748)
4, 5	5.5	(900)	7.3	(99)	7.2	(76)	5.8	(1075)
Total (N)	9.2	(1787)	11.2	(282)	10.2	(158)	9.5	(2227)
Women								
0, 1, 2	11.5	(307)	10.7	(91)	—	(28)[a]	11.9	(426)
3	6.6	(626)	11.7	(134)	2.2	(47)	7.1	(807)
4, 5	3.4	(1040)	8.4	(134)	3.3	(86)	3.9	(1260)
Total (N)	5.8	(1973)	10.3	(359)	6.0	(161)	6.4	(2493)

[a]Rates not calculated for cells with 30 or fewer individuals.

checkup even though your teeth were not giving you any trouble?" and "When was the last time you went to a doctor for a general checkup though you were feeling well and had not been sick?"

Table 3-18 shows some association between mortality and level of preventive health care. However, the health practice gradient in mortality persists through each category determined by the preventive health care index. The differences in mortality rates among health practice groups, after adjusting for age and level of preventive health care, are, again, highly significant statistically for both men and women $(P \leq .001)$. Thus although the index used may not be a very sensitive one, it does not seem that the mortality variations observed among people reporting different health practices can be accounted for by obvious differences in seeking preventive health care.

PSYCHOLOGICAL FACTORS, HEALTH PRACTICES,
AND MORTALITY

We now move to an examination of psychological variables. These are important because it is possible that psychological states or personality traits influence people to maintain high-risk behaviors. According to this idea people who are mentally disturbed, depressed, or dissatisfied with their lives are likely to maintain unhealthy habits. If this were the case, high-risk behavior could be a response to some psychological characteristic or a way in which people cope with psychological strains. It is conceivable

Table 3-18. Age-adjusted mortality rates, from all causes (per 100): Health Practices Index and level of preventive health care, men and women ages 30–69, 1965–1974

Number of low-risk health practices	Level of preventive health care							
	Low	(N)	Medium	(N)	High	(N)	Total	(N)
Men								
0, 1, 2	16.5	(223)	12.9	(116)	19.1	(65)	16.0	(404)
3	11.7	(360)	10.9	(228)	8.8	(160)	10.9	(748)
4, 5	6.4	(404)	5.8	(384)	4.8	(289)	5.8	(1077)
Total (N)	10.7	(987)	8.7	(728)	7.9	(514)	9.5	(2229)
Women								
0, 1, 2	13.6	(245)	9.2	(101)	9.4	(80)	11.9	(426)
3	7.4	(345)	8.1	(263)	5.5	(201)	7.1	(809)
4, 5	3.6	(427)	4.2	(392)	4.0	(442)	3.9	(1261)
Total (N)	7.3	(1017)	6.3	(756)	5.1	(723)	6.4	(2496)

that such psychological characteristics could be responsible for the association between health practices and mortality.

A factor analysis of the psychological variables in the 1965 survey yielded seven distinct and unidimensional factors. The factor analysis was conducted because many of the originally developed indices were of unknown validity. The description of the development of these factors and the precise items are given in the Appendix.

The cross-sectional associations between the psychological factors and health practices are generally modest. The coefficients shown in Table 3-19 from a Pearson product-moment correlation, correcting for age, are statistically significant but small, ranging from .09 to .21. For men and women the psychological scale most highly correlated with health practices is personal uncertainty. It appears that people who are unsure of themselves, or who lack some kind of directedness that allows them to make decisions, are also more likely than others to maintain high-risk health practices.

When this factor is examined in relation to the Health Practices Index and mortality rates, it is apparent that the Health Practices Index continues to predict mortality independently of the personal uncertainty factor (see Table 3-20). The differences between those scoring high and low on the Health Practices Index are statistically significant ($P \leq .001$), even though the personal uncertainty factor is associated with both mortality and health practices. For the remaining six psychological factors, age-adjusted

Table 3-19. Partial correlation coefficients (controlling for age) between Health Practices Index and psychological factors, men and women ages 30–69, 1965

Factor	Coefficient	Statistical significance
Men		
1. Personal uncertainty	−.21	.001
2. Anomy	−.12	.001
3. Life satisfaction	.13	.001
4. Social insecurity	−.09	.001
5. Perfectionism	−.06	.002
6. Negative feelings	−.14	.001
7. Isolation/depression	−.14	.001
Women		
1. Personal uncertainty	−.16	.001
2. Anomy	−.10	.001
3. Life satisfaction	.15	.001
4. Social insecurity	−.09	.001
5. Perfectionism	−.08	.001
6. Negative feelings	−.14	.001
7. Isolation/depression	−.14	.001

Table 3-20. Age-adjusted mortality rates from all causes (per 100): Health Practices Index and factor 1, personal uncertainty, men and women ages 30–69, 1965–1974

Number of low-risk health practices	Factor 1							
	High	(N)	Medium	(N)	Low	(N)	Total	(N)
Men								
0, 1, 2	18.7	(147)	16.0	(161)	11.8	(94)	15.7	(402)
3	14.2	(184)	9.6	(291)	9.6	(264)	10.7	(739)
4, 5	5.9	(181)	7.2	(372)	4.9	(517)	5.8	(1070)
Total (N)	12.8	(512)	9.8	(824)	7.3	(875)	9.4	(2211)
Women								
0, 1, 2	12.9	(191)	10.3	(140)	12.8	(93)	11.9	(424)
3	10.7	(291)	4.7	(303)	5.7	(207)	7.0	(801)
4, 5	5.2	(334)	3.4	(484)	3.8	(437)	3.9	(1255)
Total (N)	9.2	(816)	4.9	(927)	5.6	(737)	6.4	(2480)

mortality rates were also calculated and cross-tabulated with the Health Practices Index. In no case did the Health Practices Index fail to be independently associated with mortality at a highly significant level ($P \leq .001$).

Summary

The analyses have shown that common health practices are strongly associated with mortality risk among persons 30–69 years of age. Specifically, five health practices were significantly associated with mortality: (1) cigarette smoking, (2) physical activity, (3) alcohol consumption, (4) obesity, (5) sleeping patterns. Of these health practices, the first three were stronger predictors of mortality than the latter two.

To assess the cumulative impact of these five health practices, an index was developed from them. When men with 0–2 low-risk health practices were compared to men with 4 or 5 low-risk health practices, they were found to have a relative risk of dying during the follow-up period of 2.8. For women, the corresponding risk was 3.2. Without exception, for every age and sex group examined, people with high-risk health practices had higher mortality rates than those with a medium number of low-risk health practices. Those who maintained the greatest number of low-risk health practices had the lowest mortality rates.

The association between the Health Practices Index and mortality was found to be independent of a wide range of factors including self-reported physical health status at the time of the survey, year of death, socioeconomic status, race, obtaining medical and dental checkups, and many psychological factors. However, people who were in lower socio-economic groups or in poor health were from two to three times as likely to maintain high-risk health practices as those in the upper-class groups or those in better health.

References

Astrup P: Carbon monoxide, smoking and cardiovascular disease. *Circulation* 48:1167–1168, 1973.

Baekeland F, Hartmann E: Sleep requirements and the characteristics of some sleepers, in Hartmann E (ed): *Sleep and Dreaming*, International Psychiatry Clinics Series, Vol. 7. Boston, Little, Brown, 1970, pp. 33–43.

Baekeland F, Hartmann E: Reported sleep characteristics: effects of age, sleep length and psychiatric impairment. *Compr. Psychiatry* 12:141–147, 1971.

Barboriak JJ, Kory RC, Hamilton LH, Kelley FP: Changes in breakfast menu and blood lipids. *J. Am. Diet Assoc.* 49:204–206, 1966.

Bellen S, Deguzman NT, Kastic JB: The effect of inhalation of cigarette smoke on ventricular fibrillation threshold in normal dogs and dogs with acute myocardial infarction. *Am. Heart J.* **83**:67–76, 1972.

Belloc NB: Relationship of health practices and mortality. *Prev. Med.* **2**:67–81, 1973.

Belloc NB, Breslow L: Relationship of physical health status and health practices. *Prev. Med.* **1**(3):409–421, 1972.

Blackburn H, Taylor HL, Keys A: Coronary heart disease in seven countries, in Keys A (ed): *Coronary Heart Disease in Seven Countries.* New York, American Heart Association, 1970, pp. 154–211.

Brand RJ, Sholtz RI: A multiple adjustment method for combining J × 2 contingency tables for prospective and survival study analysis, paper presented at Biometrics Society Meeting, March 25, 1976.

Breslow L, Enstrom J: Persistence of health habits and their relationships to mortality. *Prev. Med.* **9**:469–483, 1980.

Brewer V, Hartmann E: Variable sleepers: when is more or less sleep required, report to the Association for the Psycho-physiological Study of Sleep, San Diego, Calif., 1973.

Build and Blood Pressure Study, 1959, Vols. I and II. Chicago, Society of Actuaries, 1959.

Cahalan C, Cisin IH: American drinking practices: summary of findings from a national probability sample. II. Measurement of massed versus spaced drinking. *Q. J. Stud. Alc.* **29**(3):642–656, 1968.

Cohn C, Joseph D: Role of rate of ingestion of diet on regulation of intermediary metabolism. *Metabolism* **9**:492–500, 1960.

Conway T, Vicker R, Ward H, Rahe R: Occupational stress and variation in cigarette, coffee and alcohol consumption. *J. Health Soc. Behav.* **22**:155–165, 1981.

Coronary Drug Project Research Group: Factors influencing long-term prognosis after recovery from myocardial infarction—three-year findings of the Coronary Drug Project. *J. Chron. Dis.* **27**:267–285, 1974.

Coronary Drug Project Research Group: Clofibrate and niacin in coronary heart disease. *J.A.M.A.* **231**(4):360–381, 1975.

Doll R, Hill AB: Mortality in relation to smoking: ten years' observations of British doctors. *Br. Med. J.* **1**:1399–1410; 1460–1467, 1964.

Enstrom JE: Cancer mortality among Mormons. *Cancer* **36**(3):825–841, 1975.

Epstein FH, Francis T, Mayner NS, et al.: Prevalence of chronic diseases and distribution of selected physiologic variables in a total community, Tecumseh, Michigan. *Am. J. Epidemiol.* **681**:307–322, 1965.

Fabry, P, Braun T: Adaptation to the pattern of food intake; some mechanisms and consequences. *Proc. Nutr. Soc.* **26**(2):144–152, 1967.

Fabry P, Tepperman J: Meal frequency—a possible factor in human pathology. *Am. J. Clin. Nutr.* **23**(8):1059–1068, 1970.

Finkelstein B, Fryer BA: Meal frequency and weight reduction of young women. *Am. J. Clin. Nutr.* **24**:465–468, 1971.

Fleiss J: *Statistical Methods for Rates and Proportions.* New York, John Wiley & Sons, 1973.

Froelicher VE: *The Effects of Chronic Exercise on the Heart and on Coronary Atherosclerotic Heart Disease; A Literature Survey.* Report SAM-TR 76-6 to the USAF School of Aerospace Medicine, February 1976.

Garn SM, Bailey SM, Cole PE, Higgins ITT: Level of education, level of income and level of fatness in adults. *Am. J. Clin. Nutr.* **30**(5):721–725, 1977.

Gordon T, Kannel WB: Predisposition to atherosclerosis in the head, heart and legs. *J.A.M.A.* **221**:661–662, 1972.

Greenspan K, Edmonds RE, Knoebel SB, et al.: Some effects of nicotine on cardiac automaticity, conduction and inotropy. *Arch. Intern. Med.* **123**:707–712, 1969.

Hammond EC: Some preliminary findings on physical complaints from a prospective study of 1,064,004 men and women. *Am. J. Public Health* **54**(1): 11–23, 1964.

Hammond EC: Smoking in relation to the death rates of one million men and women. *Natl. Cancer Inst. Monogr.* **19**:127–204, 1966.

Hammon EC, Garfinkel L: The influence of health on smoking habits. *Natl. Cancer Inst. Monogr.* **19**:269–285, 1966.

Hammond EC, Garfinkel L: Coronary heart disease, stroke, and aortic aneurysm: factors in the etiology. *Arch. Environ. Health* **19**(2):167–182, 1969.

Hartmann EL: *The Functions of Sleep*, ed 2. New Haven, Conn., Yale University Press, 1973.

Hartmann E, Baekeland F, Zwilling F, Hoy P: Sleep need: how much sleep and what kind? *Am. J. Psychiatry* **127**:1001–1008, 1971.

Hartmann E, Baekeland F, Zwilling G: Psychological differences between long and short sleepers. *Arch. Gen. Psychiatry* **26**:463–468, 1972.

Hartmann E, Galginaitis C, Moran E, Owen A, Buchanan K: When do we need more or less sleep: a study of variable sleepers, report to the 11th Annual Meeting of the Association for the Psychophysiological Study of Sleep, Lake Minnewaska, New York, Abstract in Chase M, Stern W, Walter P (eds): *Sleep Research 1971–1972*. Los Angeles, Brain Information Service, UCLA, 1972.

Haynes SG, Feinleib M, Kannel WB: The relationship of psychosocial factors to coronary heart disease in the Framingham study: eight-year incidence of coronary heart disease. *Am. J. Epidemiol.* **111**(1):37–58, 1980.

Hejda S, Fabry P: Frequency of food intake in relation to some parameters of the nutritional status. *Nutr. Dieta* **6**:215–228, 1964.

Henderson J, Enelow A: The coronary risk factor problem: a behavioral perspective. *Prev. Med.* **5**:128–148, 1976.

Hennekens CH, Willett W, Rosner B, Cole DS, Mayrent SL: Effects of beer, wine and liquor in coronary deaths. *J.A.M.A.* **242**:1973–1974, 1979.

Hennekens CH, Rosner B, Cole DS: Daily alcohol intake and coronary heart disease. *Am. J. Epidemiol.* **107**:196–200, 1978.

Heyden S, Cassel J, Bartel A, et al.: Body weight and cigarette smoking as risk factors. *Arch. Intern. Med.* **128**:915–919, 1971.

Heyman A, Karp HR, Heyden S, et al.: Cerebral vascular disease in the biracial population of Evans County. *Stroke* **2**:509–518, 1971.

Higgins MW, Kjelsberg M, Metzner H: Characteristics of smokers and nonsmokers in Tecumseh, Michigan. I. The distribution of smoking habits in persons and families and their relationship to social characteristics. *Am. J. Epidemiol.* **86**(1):45–59, 1967.

Johnson KG, Yano K, Kato H: Cerebral vascular disease in Hiroshima, Japan. *J. Chron. Dis.* **20**:545–559, 1967.

Kahn HA: The Dorn Study of smoking and mortality among U.S. veterans: report on eight and one-half years of observation. *Natl. Cancer Inst. Monogr.* **19**:1–126, 1966.

Kannel WB: Habitual level of physical activity and risk of coronary heart disease: the Framingham Study. *Can. Med. Assoc. J.* **96**:811–812, 1967.

Kannel WB: Habits and heart disease, in Palmore E, Jeffers FC (eds): *Prediction of Life Span.* Lexington, Mass, Heath Lexington Books, 1971, Chap. 5.

Kannel WB, LeBaver JE, Dawber, TR, McNamara P: Relation of body weight to development of coronary heart disease. *Circulation* **35**:734–744, 1967.

Karacan I, Thornby MA, Holzer CE, Warheit GJ, Schwab JJ, Williams RL: Prevalence of sleep disturbance in a primarily urban Florida county. *Soc. Sci. Med.* **10**:239–244, 1976.

Keys A, et al.: Coronary heart disease: overweight and obesity as risk factors. *Ann. Intern. Med.* **77**:15–27, 1972.

Khosla, T, Lowe CR: Obesity and smoking habits by social class. *Br. J. Prev. Soc. Med.* **26**:249–256, 1972.

Kissen B, Kaley MK: Alcohol and cancer, in Kissen B, Begleiter H (eds): *Alcoholism*, Vol. 34. New York, Plenum Press, 1974, pp. 481–511.

Klatsky AL, Friedman GD, Siegelaub AB: Alcohol consumption before myocardial Infarction. *Ann. Intern. Med.* **81**:294–301, 1974.

Kleitman H: *Sleep and Wakefulness*, ed 2. Chicago, University of Chicago Press, 1963.

Kripke DF, Simons RN, Garfinkel L, Hammond EC: Short and long sleep and sleeping pills: Is increased mortality associated? *Arch. Gen. Psychiatry* **36**: 103–116, 1979.

LaPorte RE, Cresanta JL, Kuller LH: The relation of alcohol to coronary heart disease and mortality: implications for public health policy. *J. Public Health Policy* **1**:198–223, 1980.

Lasserre O, Flamant R, Lellouch J, Schwartz D: Alcool et cancer: etude de pathologie geographique portant sur les departments français. *Bull. Inst. Nat. Sante* **22**:53–60, 1967.

Lemon FR, Walden RT: Death from respiratory system diseases among Seventh-Day Adventist men. *J.A.M.A.* **198**(2):137–146, 1966.

Leveille GA: Lipogenic adaptations related to pattern of food intake. *Nutr. Rev.* **30**(7):151–155, 1972a.

Leveille GA: The long-term effects of meal-eating on lipogenesis, enzyme activity, and longevity in the rat. *J. Nutr.* **102**:549–556, 1972b.

Levine PH: An acute effect of cigarette smoking on platelet function. A possible link between smoking and arterial thrombosis. *Circulation* **48**:619–623, 1973

Levinson ML: Obesity and health. *Prev. Med.* **6**(1):172–180, 1977.

Lilienfeld AM, Pedersen E, Dowd JE: *Cancer Epidemiology: Methods of Study.* Baltimore, Johns Hopkins University Press, 1967.

Lindenthal JJ, Myers JK, Pepper M: Smoking, Psychological status and stress. *Soc. Sci. Med.* **6**:583–591, 1972.

Lyon JL, Klauber MR, Gardner JW, Smart CR: Cancer incidence in Mormons and non-Mormons in Utah, 1966–1970. *N. Engl. J. Med.* **294**(3):129–133, 1976.

Mantel N. Haenszel W: Statistical aspects of the analysis of data from retrospective studies of disease. *J. Natl. Cancer Inst.* **22**:719–148, 1959.

Marmot MG, Rose G, Shipley MJ, Thomas BJ: Alcohol and mortality: a U-shaped curve. *Lancet* 1:580–583, 1981.

Metropolitan Life Insurance Company: New weight standards for men and women. *Stat. Bull. Metropol. Life Ins. Co.* 40(3):1–4, 1959.

Metropolitan Life Insurance Company: *Overweight: Its Significance and Prevention.* New York, Metropolitan Life Insurance Co., 1960.

Metzner HL, Harburg E, Lamphiear DE: Early life social incongruities, health risk factors and chronic disease. *J. Chron. Dis.* 30(4):225–245, 1977a.

Metzner H, Lamphiear N, Wheeler NC, Larkin F: The relationship between frequency of eating and adiposity in adult men and women in the Tecumseh Community Health Study. *Am. J. Clin. Nutr.* 30:712–715, 1977b.

Montoye HJ: *Physical Activity and Health: An Epidemiologic Study of an Entire Community.* Englewood Cliffs, N.J., Prentice-Hall, 1975.

Nomura A, Comstock GW, Kuller L, et al.: Cigarette smoking and strokes. *Stroke* 5:483–508, 1974.

Ostfeld AM: A review of stroke epidemiology. *Epidemiol. Rev.* 2:136–152, 1980.

Ostfeld AM, Shekelle RB, Klawans H, et al.: Epidemiology of stroke in an elderly welfare population. *Am. J. Public Health* 64:450–458, 1974.

Oswald I: The function of sleep. *Postgrad. Med. J.* 52:15–18, 1976.

Paffenbarger RS, Laughlin ME, Gima AS, Black RA: Work activity of longshoremen as related to death from coronary heart disease and stroke. *N. Engl. J. Med.* 282(20):1109–1114, 1970.

Paffenbarger RS, Wing AL: Chronic disease in former college students. XI. Early precursors of non-fatal stroke. *Am. J. Epidemiol.* 94(6):524–530, 1971.

Paffenbarger RS, Hale WE: Work activity and coronary heart mortality. *N. Engl. J. Med.* 292(11):545–550, 1975.

Paffenbarger RS, Hale WE, Brand RJ, Hyde RT: Work-energy level, personal characteristics and fatal heart atack: A birth-cohort effect. *Am J. Epidemiol.* 105(3):200–213, 1977.

Paffenbarger RS, Brand RJ, Sholtz RI, Jung DL: Energy expenditure, cigarette smoking, and blood pressure level as related to death from specific diseases. *Am. J. Epidemiol.* 108(1):12–18, 1978.

Pearson LJ: *A Study Exploring the Relationship Between Health Habit Changes, Life Change Events and Alterations in Health Status,* master's thesis, School of Nursing, University of Washington, Seattle 1974.

Pell S, D'Alonzo CA: A five-year study of alcoholics: *J. Occup. Med.* 15(2):120–125, 1973.

Phillips RL: Role of life-style and dietary habits in risk of cancer among Seventh-Day Adventists. *Cancer Res.* 35(11):3513–3522, 1975.

Phillips RL, Kuzma JW, Beeson WL, Lotz T: Influence of selection versus lifestyle on risk of fatal cancer and cardiovascular disease among Seventh-Day Adventists. *Am. J. Epidemiol.* 112(2):296–314, 1980.

Room R, Day N: Alcohol and mortality, special report to National Institute on Alcohol Abuse and Alcoholism, March 1974.

Rosenberg L, Hennekins CH, Rosner B, Belanger C, Rothman K, Speizer F: Oral contraceptive use in relation to nonfatal myocardial infarction. *Am. J. Epidemiol.* 111(1):59–66, 1980.

Rothman KJ: Alcohol, in Fraumeni J. (ed): *Persons at High Risk of Cancer: An*

Approach to Cancer Etiology and Control. New York, Academic Press, 1975, pp. 139–150.

Schmidt W: Effects of alcohol consumption on health. *J. Public Health Policy* 1:25–40, 1980.

Schmidt W, DeLint J: Causes of death of alcoholics. *Q. J. Stud. Alc.* 33(1):171–185, 1972.

Schwartz D, Lasserre O, Flamant R, Lellouch J: Alcool et cancer: etude de pathologie geographique portant sur 19 pays. *Eur. J. Cancer* 2:367–372, 1966.

Selikoff IJ, Hammond EC, Churg J: Asbestos exposure, smoking and neoplasia. *J.A.M.A.* 204:106–112, 1968.

Stamler J, Lindberg HA, Berkson DM, Shaffer A, Miller W, Poindexter A: Prevalence and incidence of coronary heart disease in strata of the labor force of a Chicago industrial corporation. *J. Chron. Dis.* 11(4):405–420, 1960.

Stason W, Neff R, Miettinen O, Jick H: Alcohol consumption and nonfatal myocardial infarction. *Am. J. Epidemiol.* 104:603–608, 1976.

Stunkard A, et al.: Influence of social class on obesity and thinness in children. *J.A.M.A.* 221:579, 1972.

Tepperman J, Brobeck JR, Long C: The effects of hypothalmic hyperphagia and of alteration of feeding habits on the metabolism of the albino rat. *Yale J. Biol. Med.* 15:855–874, 1943.

United States, Dept. of Health, Education and Welfare, Public Health Service, Division of Chronic Diseases, Heart Disease Control Program: Health implications, in *Obesity and Health—A Source Book of Current Information for Public Health Personnel,* Publ. NO.1485, Washington, D.C., U.S. Government Printing Office, 1966.

United States, Dept. of Health, Education and Welfare, Public Health Service, Center for Disease Control: *The Health Consequences of Smoking—1975.* Washington, D.C., U.S. Government Printing Office, 1975.

United States, Dept. of Health, Education and Welfare, Public Health Service, National Institute on Alcohol Abuse and Alcoholism: *Alcohol and Health, New Knowledge.* Washington, D.C., U.S. Government Printing Office, 1975.

Wadhwa PS, Young EA, Schmidt K, Elson CE, Pringle DJ: Metabolic consequences of feeding frequency in man. *Am. J. Clin. Nutr.* 26:823–830, 1973.

Webb WB, Agnew HW, Jr.: Sleep stage characteristics of long and short sleepers. *Science* 168:146–147, 1970.

Wiley, JA, Camacho TC: Life style and future health: evidence from the Alameda County study. *Prev. Med.* 9:1–21, 1980.

World Health Organization: Smoking and disease: the evidence reviewed. *WHO Chron.* 29:402–408, 1975.

Wynder EL, Bross IJ: Aetiological factors in mouth cancer. *Br. Med. J.* 1:1137–1143, May 18, 1957.

Wynder EL, Lemon FR, Bross IJ: Cancer and coronary artery disease among Seventh-Day Adventists. *Cancer* 12(5):1016–1028, 1959.

Wynder EL, Mabuchi K: Etiological and preventive aspects of human cancer. *Prev. Med.* 1:300–334, 1972.

Yano K, Rhoads GG, Kagan A, Tillotson J: Dietary intake and the risk of coronary heart disease in Japanese men living in Hawaii. *Am. J. Clin. Nutr.* **31**:1270–1279, 1978.

Young CM, Frankel DL, Scanlan SS, Simko V, Lutwak L: Frequency of feeding, weight reduction, and nutrient utilization. *J. Am. Diet. Assoc.* **59**(5):473–480, 1971a.

Young CM, Scanlan SS, Topping CM, Simko V, Lutwak L: Frequency of feeding, weight reduction, and body composition. *J. Am. Diet. Assoc.* **59**(5):466–472, 1971b.

Young CM, Hutter LF, Scanlan SS, Rand CE, Lutwak L, Simko V: Metabolic effects of meal frequency on normal young men. *J. Am. Diet. Assoc.* **61**:391–398, 1972.

4. Social networks and mortality risk

Although the social environment obviously exerts some effect on health, precisely which features of that environment are deleterious is not so clear. Numerous studies have shown associations between health status and social disorganization, rapid social change, social class, marital status, occupational mobility and strain, ethnicity, and geographic mobility. These studies have given rise to the notion of socioenvironmental stress in which specific changes or "life events," such as job change, death of a spouse, and divorce, appear to be stressful and thus potentially disease producing. Typified in the work of Holmes and Rahe, who developed scales for indicating the relative importance of these life events, such occurrences are often seen as increasing the risk of illness because they deplete a person's "adaptive energy" or because they arouse debilitating alarm and distress reactions.

Research along this line has proceeded rapidly, and measurement of life changes has become quite sophisticated. Viewing socioenvironmental stress as a predominantly acute phenomenon has limitations, however, the most troublesome of which is that only modest correlations exist between acute events and subsequent illness. Apparently some people experiencing stressful events become ill, but many others do not seem to experience any health changes at all (Mueller et al., 1977; Rabkin and Struening, 1976). In addition, although acutely stressful situations may cause transient physiological changes, minor illnesses, or exacerbations of preexisting conditions, the evidence does not as clearly show that acute stressors induce more serious chronic or disabling conditions (Dohrenwend and Dohrenwend, 1978; Theorell et al., 1975). Finally, though a stressful event is by definition an acute phenomenon, it may exert a lasting effect by changing one's ability to cope with circumstances or by altering one's social milieu. Death of a spouse, for instance, which is included in most Holmes and Rahe-type scales, also has long-lasting consequences by creating the "condition" of widowhood. Viewing such a death as merely a short episode may obscure the possibly enduring effects of widowhood.

Some investigators have therefore begun to examine long-standing stressful situations in the social environment. Certain occupational demands and working conditions, and poverty exemplify this latter kind of chronic stress. Lazarus and Cohen (1976) have suggested that "chronic hassles," which involve dealing with difficult situations on a daily basis, may be more taxing on one's adaptive energy than short-term situations.

The role of social networks in health

On the other hand, evidence is mounting that some factors in the social milieu protect health and well-being. Foremost among these are the kinds of social ties a person maintains with other individuals and the community at large. These social networks provide a web that seems to assure every person in it of receiving a certain amount of emotional and practical support. With strong social support, even someone who is experiencing difficulties does not suffer to the same extent as a more isolated individual. Social networks and their association with health are the focus of this chapter.

We will examine the ties that people have to one another, the characteristics of these ties, and how they relate to health. It should be noted that this approach does not concentrate on the attributes of people in the network but rather on the social linkages of one person to another (Mitchell, 1969; Whitten and Wolfe, 1974). Thus we do not consider whether an individual is "antisocial" or lonely, but whether he or she reports contacts with friends or relatives, and the quality of those relationships. This kind of analysis, frequently called Social Network Analysis, seems to offer a useful approach to understanding disease risk from the social environment.

First, the search for factors in the social environment that may be associated with increased disease risk has brought attention to such varied groups as migrants, widows, those in lower social classes, and those undergoing rapid social change. It would seem useful, then, to examine conditions that are common to such high-risk social groups. One characteristic of people in these groups is that they have comparatively few social and community ties and resources (Bell and Boat, 1957; Bell and Force, 1965; Berkman, 1977; Litwak, 1960).

Second, social networks are important to consider because they are intertwined with life events or changes. Several reviews of this relationship point in the same direction (Berkman, 1981; Mueller, 1980; Thoits, 1982). Many life changes, in fact the ones most consistently associated with poor health, consist of breaks in social ties such as death of a spouse, divorce, or marital separation. Life event checklists often include items such as trouble with co-workers or spouse, which imply something about the quality of networks and represent long-standing situations, rather than discrete occurrences.

Another possibility is that social networks are antecedent to and influence the occurrence of major life changes. A study of how people find jobs indicated that the majority of people who found a job through an acquaintance saw that acquaintance occasionally, not often, and not rarely (Granovetter, 1973). Goldberg and Comstock (1980), exploring the relationship between life events and demographic characteristics, reported that married people are less likely than the single, widowed, divorced, or separated to report five or more such happenings in a one-year period. These data suggest that the frequency of life changes may be determined in part by network structures.

Furthermore, many events may seriously "disrupt, distort, reduce, or otherwise change existing network relationships" (Mueller, 1980). Moving, changing jobs, or retiring almost inevitably causes changes in social relationships. Mueller (1980) has suggested that much of the impact of such occurrences "may result from the profound disturbances they introduce into one's social network." As yet there are no data with which to address this issue.

Finally, it is possible that social networks are coping resources that enable an individual to avoid the deleterious consequences of life change. The extent to which an individual maintains social support in certain situations may profoundly affect (1) the way the situation is ultimately resolved and (2) the emotional impact of the situation on the individual. These, in turn, may influence the degree to which the event has serious health consequences. Some data, in fact, link these phenomena.

In a study of the mental and physical health consequences of job loss because of a factory shutdown, Gore (1978) reported that those unemployed for several weeks who had the emotional support of their spouses experienced few symptoms of illness, had low cholesterol levels, and did not blame themselves for the job loss.

Social networks seem to play a similar role in helping bereaved people adjust to widowhood. McKinlay (1980) has suggested that social networks, more than any other variable, may determine how a person copes with the death of a loved one. Other investigators have noted that various kinds of network ties are important at different times in the bereavement process (Walker et al., 1977). Soon after the death, grieving persons need emotional support, which is best supplied by close friends and relatives. Later, however, the widow or widower must move on to a new life and look to the future. During these subsequent phases of adjustment, people with whom the bereaved person has less intimate or weaker ties may facilitate adjustment by supplying new information and sources of contact. These weaker ties may then be more useful to the bereaved person than closer, more emotionally important ties.

Occupational stress differs from the life events just discussed, but because it is a chronically stressful situation, here too social support may be a buffer. In a study of NASA professionals, Caplan (1971) found little relationship between occupational stress and heart disease risk among men reporting high levels of support from their co-workers. Among those without support, a significant association did exist.

House and Wells (1978), in a cross-sectional study of 1809 men working in a manufacturing plant, examined the effect of social support from supervisors, co-workers, friends, relatives, and wives on job stress and on physical and mental health. Support appeared to lessen the impact of perceived job stresses and their subsequent impact on health. This influence was more apparent in some self-reported health outcomes, such as ulcers and neurotic symptoms, than in others—for example, angina pectoris, itching and rash, cough and phlegm. The support of supervisors and wives was more beneficial than that of co-workers, friends, and relatives. The buffer effect of support may be explained by the fact that the items measuring social support emphasized respondents' perceptions of emotional supportiveness concerning mostly work-related problems. Thus the social support was specific to the particular stress being studied and would not be expected to have an impact on health in the absence of job stress.

Social networks may thus decrease the health impact of life events or chronic stress. They may also significantly affect health apart from such situations. Evidence of the direct health effects of social networks is just beginning to accumulate and will be reviewed in two parts: (1) the effects of intimate ties and (2) the effects of other social and community ties.

The health effects of intimate ties

Marriage obviously is one of the most fundamental and intimate ties between people. Those who are not married, whether single, separated, widowed, or divorced, experience higher mortality rates than married people (Carter and Glick, 1970; Ortmeyer, 1974; Thiel et al., 1973). These differences cannot be explained by an increase in any one cause of death (Ortmeyer, 1974). Divorced white men have higher mortality rates than their married counterparts for virtually every major cause of death except leukemia. That is also true of single white men, with the added exception of malignant neoplasms of genital organs. Compared to married men, those who are single have a mortality rate that is four times higher from cancer of the digestive organs and peritoneum. Widowed men have seven times the homicide rate, four times the suicide rate, and over six times the mortality rate for tuberculosis and cirrhosis of the liver. Divorced white women experience higher death rates from almost all causes compared with those who are married; and single white women have higher rates than married white women for most causes. The cause-specific ratios are not as great for women, however, as they are for men.

Widowhood profoundly affects mental and physical well-being (Cox and Ford, 1964; Kraus and Lilienfeld, 1959; Maddison and Viola, 1968; Marris, 1958; McNeil, 1973; Parkes, 1964; Rees and Lutkins, 1967). For example, Parkes, Benjamin, and Fitzgerald (1969) found that 4486 widowers 55 years of age and older, during the first 6 months after the death of their wives, experienced a mortality rate 40 percent above that expected for married men the same age. The greatest excess in mortality occurred among widowers who died of coronary thrombosis and other arteriosclerotic disease, although increased risk was observed for many causes of death.

In a comprehensive and well-controlled analysis of widowhood, Helsing et al. (1981) found that being a widow or widower carried an increased mortality risk among men, but not among women. Their 10-year retrospective-cohort study of men and women in Washington County, Maryland, showed that the excessive risk in men persisted when age, education, age at first marriage, cigarette smoking, church attendance, and a proxy economic status measure were controlled. In contrast to other investigators, Helsing and co-workers reported that the increased mortality risk among widowers was not confined to the first 6 months of the bereavement but persisted throughout a 10-year follow-up period. If further studies confirm this finding, it would seem reasonable to view widowhood as a chronically stressful situation or social condition rather than attributing the increased mortality to the acute effects of the spouse's death (Helsing and Szklo, 1981; Susser, 1981).

Socioeconomic status conceivably could account for mortality rate differences between married and unmarried people. Both the British study by Parkes et al. (1969) and the study by Helsing and Szklo (1981), however, disclosed increased mortality risks for widowers when socioeconomic status was controlled. Also, a Finnish study with control for social class indicates that mortality from ischemic heart disease is higher among divorced and widowed persons (Koskenvuo et al., 1980).

Attempting to understand what might account for the increased risk of dying from coronary heart disease (CHD) among unmarried people, Weiss (1973) examined the relationship between marital status, CHD, serum cholesterol, systolic and diastolic blood pressure, and ponderal index in a sample of 6672 adults interviewed in the U.S. Health Examination Survey. He found substantial CHD risks associated with being single, widowed, or divorced, but no consistent differences in the traditional risk factors between married and unmarried men and women. Some evidence to the contrary, however, has come from Finland where A. Aromaa reported that married men smoke less than other men and have lower systolic and diastolic blood pressure than widowed men, and that divorced women smoke more than married women ("Social Insurance Coronary Heart Disease Study," unpublished data, reviewed in Koskenvuo et al., 1980).

Having either a supportive partner or a spouse may buffer the impact of stressful events. In a study of 220 urban women, Brown and colleagues (1975) found that having a husband or boyfriend who was a confidant seemed to afford protection against the onset of depression in the presence of mounting life changes. Of those with many life events but with no supportive partner, 38% reported depression; on the other hand, only 4% of those experiencing serious life disturbances with a confiding relationship— husband or boyfriend—developed depression. Lowenthal and Haven have reported the significance among the elderly of having a confidant (1967).

The health effects of extended family, friends, and community ties

Most people rely on brothers, sisters, aunts, uncles, parents, friends, work associates, and neighbors to fulfill a variety of emotional and practical needs. Besides enduring and close relationships, some of these connections seem weaker and largely task-oriented. Taken as a whole, these enduring relationships and informal associations form a web in which most people spend a significant portion of their lives. Although several social scientists have described such network configurations in detail (Bott, 1971; Fischer et al., 1977; Laumann, 1973; Mitchell, 1969), relatively little is known about their impact on health status.

Social networks appear to play an important role in pregnancy out-comes. For example, a study of primipara army wives disclosed that those with many life changes but rich psychosocial resources had only one-third the complication rate of women in similar circumstances but with few psychosocial resources (Nuckolls et al., 1972). In this study, social networks and many other psychosocial factors were included in one psychosocial asset score, prohibiting the assessment of the impact of networks alone on pregnancy outcomes. In two other studies, networks evidently affected the complications of delivery (Sosa et al., 1980) and postpartum emotional problems (Gordon and Gordon, 1967). In the latter study, the absence of supportive family and friends predisposed women to postpartum depression.

Social networks have also been reported to play a role in compliance and efficacy of treatment regimens. DeAraujo et al. (1973) found the Berle Index, a composite measure of psychosocial resources including family and interpersonal relationships, to be negatively associated with steroid requirements of asthma patients. People who report not having enough friends (Segal et al., 1967) or those who are weakly integrated into a new society (Shuval et al., 1970) apparently use health services in general to a greater extent than others. Withdrawal from alcohol and compliance with medical regimes both appear linked with social support, according to a review by Cobb (1976). A review of 22 studies of compliance and social support by Haynes and Sackett (1974) revealed that 15 of them suggested a relationship of social support with compliance to therapeutic regimes; one study produced evidence to the contrary and six studies showed no difference. Many investigators have examined social support in relation to coping with severe illness, and to recovery and rehabilitation (Croog and Levine, 1972; Doehrman, 1977; Hyman, 1972; Litman, 1966).

The research presented thus far has tended to focus on strong ties, particularly with close friends and family, which are characterized by emotional intensity, intimacy, and reciprocity. However, other network analyses indicate the importance and cohesive power of what have been called "weak ties" (Granovetter, 1973). Although typically lacking intimacy and with limited time spent in the relationship, these ties, Granovetter argues, may facilitate the diffusion of influence and information, and provide opportunities for mobility and for political and community organization. Walker, MacBride, and Vachon (1977) suggest that weak ties help bereaved people at a time when they need new information and new contacts. Other studies indicate that differentiated networks or more varied types of contact may aid access to medical care (Lee, 1969; McKinlay, 1973). Spouses of people with such networks tend to recover more successfully from heart attacks (Finlayson, 1976). Closely knit networks in which most people in the network know each other may provide strong emotional support but may be limiting in their support by reducing access to information and resources. When the dominant in-group values and beliefs are incompatible with appropriate preventive behavior or seeking medical care, closed networks may be associated with poorer health status. Suchman (1966) has analyzed this issue.

The relationship between nonintimate, weak ties and health status has not been thoroughly investigated. Most research in this area has been limited to studying group affiliations, organizational memberships, and social participation, instead of directly measuring extended ties. Joseph (1980) conducted one study of social affiliations, in relation to coronary heart disease among Japanese-Americans in California. A sample of 3809 Japanese-American men aged 30–74 in the San Francisco Bay area was studied to ascertain the association between acculturation, biologic risk factors, and CHD (Marmot and Syme, 1976; Nichaman et al., 1975; Winkelstein et al., 1975). Joseph examined the cross-sectional relationships between degree of social affiliation, biologic risk factors, and prevalence of CHD. By including mild cases, probable as well as definite CHD, Joseph reduced the bias that severe illness might have on patterns or reports of social affiliation. Her multiple logistic risk analysis of physical risk factors (serum cholesterol, systolic blood pressure, cigarette smoking, family history of heart attack, and physical activity) and social affiliation (marital status, attendance at religious services, and membership in either formal or informal organizations) showed that social affiliation, age, physical inactivity, and family history of heart attack were independently associated with the prevalence of coronary heart disease. When the extreme categories of low to high social affiliation were compared, the approximate relative risk was 1.94.

The long-established association of church attendance with mental and physical health conceivably could result from religious belief, health-related behavior associated with religious belief, health status, social and demographic factors, or support provided by a church group. Compared with people who attend church infrequently, churchgoers respond more favorably to cervical cancer screening programs (Naguib et al., 1968). The latter also have a lower risk of arteriosclerotic heart disease, pulmonary emphysema, suicide, cirrhosis of the liver, high blood pressure, and tuberculosis (Comstock and Partridge, 1972; Comstock et al., 1970; Graham et al., 1978). Seventh-Day Adventists and Mormons maintain comparatively good health status, presumably explained in part by their favorable health behaviors such as avoidance of tobacco and alcohol. An Israeli study documented a lower incidence of myocardial infarction among the more religious Jews (Medalie et al. 1973).

The wealth of data on social networks and mental health are of variable quality. At least three reviews have been published recently (Dean and Lin, 1977; Mueller, 1980; Thoits, 1982). For the most part, research in this area supports the notion that social networks interact with life experiences to decrease symptoms of psychological distress.

Phillips (1967) found that people who have frequent contacts with friends, neighbors, or organizational associates report "being happy" more often and are less likely to score "impaired" on Langner's Psychiatric Scale than those with infrequent contacts. In a random sample of 142 adults in Canberra, Australia, Henderson et al. (1978) found a strong inverse relationship between social bonds and the presence of neurotic symptoms. In a larger study, with control for adverse life events, Henderson (1978a) confirmed these findings and showed a statistically significant decline in symptoms with increasing strength of social bonds. A study by Wechsler and Pugh (1967) of approximately 25,000 first admissions to Massachusetts mental hospitals provided an indirect test of the role of extended ties. The investigators hypothesized that any difference between an individual's demographic characteristics and those of others in his community would indicate the availability of a peer group for interpersonal relationships. People dissimilar to others in the community with respect to age, marital, status, occupation, and place of birth experienced higher than expected rates of hospital admissions.

These studies, taken as a whole, suggest that social networks influence the development of physical and mental illness. However, many questions remain in the absence of data on the association between networks and disease incidence, and very little is known about the network relationship (other than marital status) to mortality.

A troublesome question is whether prior illness determines social network configurations rather than the reverse. Because much work on the matter has been cross-sectional or without adequate control for health status, this possibility must be examined in detail.

Another question is how social networks are physiologically linked to disease. Research to date has shown that social networks are associated with diverse health outcomes, suggesting multiple biologic pathways from networks to illness and/or that social isolation leads to decreased resistance to disease in general.

From the literature, what it is about networks that may be important to health is not clear. The data published so far do not show whether the quality of relationship is more significant than the quantity of contacts, whether intimate ties are more related than extended ones, or whether cumulative effects occur with increasing isolation.

Data from the Human Population Laboratory

Considerations outlined in the preceding section prompted us to analyze the Human Population Laboratory data concerning social networks and their possible relationship to mortality. The 1965 survey included several items on the nature and degree of social contacts. Originally included in the questionnaire to measure social well-being, these items conform well to network measures used in sociological and epidemiologic work. The questionnaire covered four kinds of social contacts: (1) marriage, (2) contacts with extended family and close friends, (3) church membership, and (4) other group affiliations. Information was thus available on both intimate contacts (marriage and close friends and relatives) and more extended or weaker ties (church and group affiliations). This provided an opportunity to compare different types of contacts and their possible cumulative impact.

Most previous investigators had focused on either intimate ties *or* broad social affiliations. The main limitation of HPL data for social network measures is that they only crudely indicate the potential array of links an individual has with others. This is especially true of extended ties. Also, the data only minimally reflect the quality of relationships. Some items bear on satisfaction in marriage, but the survey in general elicited little about a particular relationship and whether it was meeting emotional or instrumental needs.

On the other hand, the HPL questionnaire did incorporate information about other factors known to be related to morbidity and mortality (smoking, obesity, alcohol consumption, and other health practices; use of health services; socioeconomic status), and to social networks (mobility, socioeconomic status, psychological states). This permits analyses in which many potentially confounding factors can be taken into account.

In this chapter we analyze social networks, as measured in the baseline survey in 1965, for their prediction of mortality throughout the 9-year follow-up period. The networks are examined individually and then cumulatively in a Social Network Index. Whether several other factors might account for any association between social networks and mortality is then investigated. The two subsequent chapters provide further analyses of the relationship. Chapter 5 consists of a multiple logistic analysis of mortality and social networks, health practices, physical health status, and other demographic variables. Chapter 6 presents data on how social networks and health practices are related to changes in health status between 1965 and 1974.

Marital status

Data from the Human Population Laboratory support previous findings of a relationship between marital status and mortality from all causes. As seen in Table 4-1, people 30–69 years of age who were married had lower

Table 4-1. Age-adjusted mortality rates from all causes (per 100): types of social contact, men and women ages 30–69, 1965–1974

Type of social contact	30–49 yrs. No.	30–49 yrs. %Died	50–59 yrs. No.	50–59 yrs. %Died	60–69 yrs. No.	60–69 yrs. %Died	P value[a] for χ^2
Men							
Marital status							
Married	1227	3.0	446	12.1	268	26.9	
Unmarried	175	8.6	55	25.5	98	33.7	$P \le .001$
Contacts with friends and relatives							
High	276	2.9	127	11.0	81	22.2	
Medium	865	3.4	303	14.2	173	24.9	$P \le .001$
Low	236	5.1	62	14.5	59	40.7	
Church membership							
Member	391	2.8	168	11.3	88	21.6	
Nonmember	1011	4.1	333	14.7	238	30.3	$P \le .05$
Group membership							
Member	1066	3.6	394	11.9	223	28.2	
Nonmember	336	3.9	107	19.6	103	27.2	n.s.[b]
Women							
Marital status							
Married	1249	3.0	407	7.1	208	14.4	
Unmarried	286	3.8	167	9.6	179	20.7	n.s.
Contacts with friends and relatives							
High	266	1.9	166	6.6	105	11.4	
Medium	1007	2.9	340	7.6	223	17.0	$P \le .001$
Low	239	5.4	57	12.3	41	31.0	
Church membership							
Member	484	1.4	217	6.9	152	15.8	
Nonmember	1051	3.9	357	8.4	235	18.3	$P \le .05$
Group membership							
Member	1005	2.4	347	7.2	173	15.0	
Nonmember	535	4.5	227	8.8	214	19.2	$P \le .05$

[a]Chi-square values were calculated for differences in age-adjusted mortality rates among categories.
[b]n.s., Not significant.

mortality rates than those who were separated, widowed, single, and divorced. The relative risk for unmarried women compared to married women is approximately 1.4 throughout the age range studied. For men the relative risk of being unmarried was greater at the younger ages, especially 30–49 years when the relative risk was nearly 3. The age-adjusted chi-square value for the differences in mortality rates among men of different marital status is highly significant; for women, the same chi square fails to reach statistical significance.

These findings confirm previous observations that not being married imposes a greater health risk on men than on women. Based on a study of suicide rates, Durkheim (1951) theorized that the institution of marriage was more beneficial to men than to women. Upon the dissolution of marriage, men lost not only a marriage but frequently a family social group, whereas women lost a conjugal association, which had held some benefits, but generally retained a family, which had many more. Increased mortality among widowed men but not widowed women has been previously noted (Helsing et al., 1981; Susser, 1981).

If marriage itself is a protective factor for health, then one can hypothesize further that people who are satisfied and happy with their marriage would have better health, expressed in lower mortality rates, than those who experience more conflict in marriage. The Human Population Laboratory provided an opportunity to test this hypothesis with a marital adjustment index composed of nine questions including whether or not an individual receives understanding from the spouse, has thought about getting a divorce or separation, or has had many problems in a marriage. The items comprising the index appear in the Appendix, p, 233. They provide a subjective rating or marital adjustment with emphasis on whether emotional needs are being met. Figure 4-1 shows age- and sex-specific mortality rates for three levels of marital satisfaction. For women, no clear pattern is discernible; if anything, the more satisfied women over 50 appeared to have less favorable mortality rates. Among men 30–59 years of age, those who reported satisfaction and few problems with their marriage in 1965 had lower mortality rates than the men with more difficulties in their marriages. This association is not evident for men 60–69 years of age. The chi-square value, adjusted for age, is not significant ($P \geq .05$) for either men or women.

Of course, the measure of the quality of marital relationships used here may not be a good one. For example, the social desirability of reporting one's marriage to be happy may have caused poor classification. If the index is an adequate measure of interactional quality, however, then these data suggest that a marital tie itself rather than the quality of the relationship carries an impact on mortality. Further work is needed to assess more adequately the relative importance of quality versus quantity in social contacts. Marriage was the only relationship for which information on quality of contact was available from the 1965 survey.

Close friends and relatives

Although it is commonly held that extended family and close friends can buffer stressful situations and protect the individual against serious social

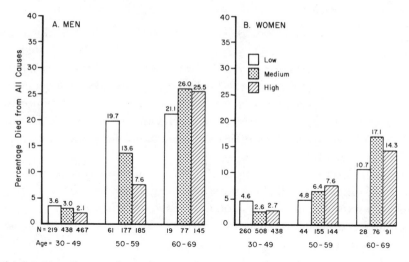

Fig. 4-1. Mortality rates from all causes: marital adjustment index, age- and sex-specific rates, 1965–1974.

and psychological losses, relatively little is known about the impact of these relationships on health. In order to examine whether having close friends and relatives may affect mortality, HPL investigators devised an index of such relationships. It consisted of three questions in the 1965 survey: (1) How many close friends do you have? (2) How many relatives do you have that you feel close to? (3) How often do you see these people each month?

Although individually these items were not powerful predictors of mortality, when combined into the index they did indicate significant increases in risk of dying. Table 4-1 shows that for every age and sex category examined, people who scored low on the index experienced higher mortality rates than those who scored high. The age-adjusted chi-square values for both men and women are highly significant ($P \leq .001$).

It is of interest that differences in mortality rates between people who score high and low on the friends and relatives index are greater for women than for men. The relative risks are 1.3–1.8 for men, but for women in the age groups studied, the relative risks are 1.9–2.8. Thus it appears that whereas marital status is a stronger predictor of mortality among men, having contacts with friends and relatives may have a greater effect among women. Furthermore, for both men and women, it was only the absence of both friends and relatives that resulted in a significantly increased mortality risk.

Church membership

Beyond marriage, and close friends and relatives, membership in an organization provides social connections that may be related to health. The HPL survey contained several items concerning membership in both formal and informal groups, specifically whether an individual belonged to any social or recreational group, labor union, commercial or professional association, church, group concerned with children such as PTA or Boy Scouts, any service group, charity, community-betterment group, or any other organization.

If membership in these groups provides an important source of contacts, one might expect that people who belong to them would have lower mortality rates than people who do not belong to such groups. To investigate this hypothesis, two analyses were done. In one, church membership was examined separately; in the other, membership in one or more groups other than church was examined. Church membership may be regarded as conceptually different from other types of associations. Also, because previous research had suggested that church attendance is related to health, it seemed important to test this hypothesis separately.

The results corroborate previous findings that individuals who belong to a church have a better health record than those who do not. Table 4-1 shows that for every sex and age group examined, individuals who belong to a church experience lower mortality than those who do not. The differences are not as large as those observed in the case of marital status or friends and relatives, but they are consistent. The greatest difference in mortality rates between church members and nonmembers appears in women 30–49 years of age: a relative risk approaching 3. In other age and sex groups the relative risks do not exceed 1.5. The age-adjusted chi-square values are statistically significant $(P \leq .05)$ for both men and women.

Group membership

Membership in other than church groups was similarly related to mortality. With the exception of men 60–69 years old, both men and women who belonged to one or more formal and informal groups had lower mortality rates than individuals who did not belong to any groups. Table 4-1 indicates that the greatest differential is again among the youngest women. Although the differences for men are not significant $(P \geq .05)$, they are significant for women $(P = .02)$.

Group membership does not appear to predict mortality as strongly as more intimate contacts such as in marriage or with close friends and relatives. In no case do the age- and sex-specific relative risks between those who are and those who are not members of nonchurch groups exceed 2 and, in most cases, they are not over 1.5.

The cumulative impact of social networks

Mortality rates thus show gradients with respect to marital status, contact with close friends, church membership, and affiliation with other groups. The next step was to examine how these kinds of social ties interacted with one another in order to assess their cumulative effects on mortality. For this purpose a Social Network Index was constructed, comparable to the Health Practices Index presented in Chapter 3. The Social Network Index was intended to provide a convenient way of examining associations among social networks, mortality, and other possibly related variables. Essentially, the analyses conducted for the health practices were repeated for social networks. Also, in Chapter 5 the independence of each of the four components of the Social Network Index are assessed using the multiple logistic approach.

An interesting question is whether people can substitute one type of contact for another and still maintain low mortality risk. As noted earlier in this chapter, whether contacts are among friends or relatives does not seem important; it is only when both are absent that a significant increase in death rate occurs. Similarly, people who were not married but had many friends and relatives experienced mortality rates comparable to those who were married but had few contacts with friends and relatives, as shown in Table 4-2. According to these data, no single social relation-

Table 4-2. Age-adjusted mortality rates from all causes (per 100): index of friends and relatives and marital status, men and women ages 30–69, 1965–1974

Friends and relatives index	Marital status					
	Not married	(N)	Married	(N)	Total	(N)
Men						
Low	16.3	(67)	11.6	(290)	12.5	(357)
Medium	16.7	(178)	8.1	(1210)	9.2	(1388)
High	6.6	(43)	7.6	(441)	7.4	(484)
Total (N)	14.7	(288)	8.4	(1941)	9.5	(2229)
Women						
Low	9.5	(87)	12.0	(251)	11.2	(338)
Medium	8.0	(405)	5.5	(1216)	6.2	(1621)
High	6.4	(140)	3.5	(397)	4.6	(537)
Total (N)	7.6	(632)	5.8	(1864)	6.4	(2496)

ship is totally responsible for the association between mortality and social networks; for example, both marital status and close friends and relatives are independently related to that risk.

Furthermore, when these close ties were examined in relation to more extended connections to church and other groups, both types of social relationships predicted mortality but the former were more powerful predictors. The data also revealed cumulative effects associated with social networks, indicating that the sheer quantity of contacts may be an important determinant of mortality risk. Only in the presence of severe social disconnection, when an individual has few links in any sphere of interaction, do mortality rates rise sharply. In general, it appears that people can trade off or substitute one source of contact for another and still maintain a reasonably low mortality risk.

To summarize the effects on mortality of increasing social isolation, a Social Network Index was constructed based on the four kinds of contacts categorized in Table 4-1. The index includes both the number of social ties and their relative importance. Thus intimate contacts are weighted more heavily than church and other group affiliations.

Figure 4-2 displays the distribution of scores on the Social Network Index in various age and sex groups. Approximately one-tenth of persons 30–69 years of age fall into the most isolated category. Among men of different ages, no major differences in network scores are observed. Among women, however, those 60–69 years of age tend to be more isolated than younger women. Sex differences are not large; women fall

Fig. 4-2. Age and sex distribution of Social Network Index scores, 1965.

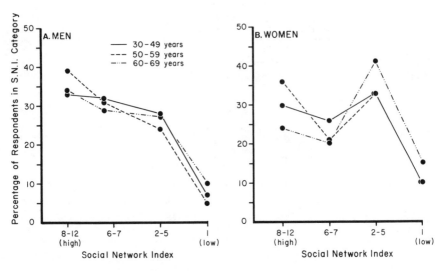

somewhat lower on the Social Network Index, partly because of their greater likelihood of being divorced, separated, or widowed.

Figure 4-3, displaying the age- and sex-specific mortality rates for the Social Network Index, shows the consistent pattern of higher mortality rates with each decrease in social connection. The only exception appears among women aged 50–59. The relative risks of those most isolated compared to those with most social connections are shown at the base of the figure. For men in various age groups the relative risks range from 1.8 to 3.2; for women, 2.1 to 4.6. The age-adjusted relative risks are 2.3 for men and 2.8 for women ($P \leq .001$).

The mortality risks associated with scoring low on the Social Network Index are greater than those associated with any single network measure or with intimate contacts, suggesting some cumulative effect. It should be noted, however, that the index is weighted by intimate contacts, reflecting both quality (intimate versus extended) and quantity of social contact.

Do inadequate social networks result in fatal illness or vice versa?

Clearly, the extent of people's social networks is associated with their mortality rates. One possible explanation implied throughout this chapter is that the existence of strong social ties reduces the risk of premature death. Equally conceivable is the hypothesis that people who are sick and likely to die soon may be unable to maintain social ties. Accordingly, illness may precede and "cause" the social disconnection, not the reverse. This is a difficult issue to assess, but two separate attempts were made to ascertain the direction of influence.

First, if physical illness at the time of the 1965 survey were responsible for the social disconnection reported, it would be expected that such seriously ill people would die mostly in the early years following the survey. Table 4-3 shows, however, that only a small proportion of the deaths among social isolates occurred during the first 2 years. In fact, the percentage of deaths occurring in the first years after the survey was the same among isolated and connected groups. Although the figures in this table are not age-adjusted, other analyses indicate that social networks are associated with mortality independently of age.

A second approach to the problem was to examine the relationship between networks and mortality while controlling for level of physical health in 1965. An index of physical health had been developed and used for the 1965 survey data, with acceptable reliability and validity (Hochstim and Renne, 1971). The index, called the Physical Health Spectrum and described in Chapter 2, assigns people to four categories: (1) those re-

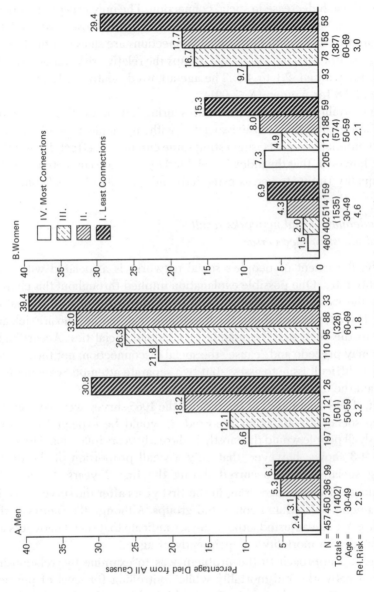

Fig. 4-3. Mortality from all causes: Social Network Index, age- and sex-specific rates (per 100), 1965–1974.

Table 4-3. Percentage of deaths occurring by year of death and Social Network Index, men and women ages 30–69, 1965–1974

Social Network Index[a]	Year of death											
	1965–1966		1967–1968		1969–1970		1971–1972		1973–1974		Total deaths	
	%	(N)	%	(N)	%	(N)	%	(N)	%	(N)	%	(N)
Men												
I	15	(4)	26	(7)	26	(7)	18	(5)	15	(4)	100	(27)
II	19	(14)	18	(13)	21	(15)	21	(15)	21	(15)	100	(72)
III	16	(9)	19	(11)	17	(10)	32	(19)	16	(9)	100	(58)
IV	15	(8)	19	(10)	19	(10)	27	(15)	20	(11)	100	(54)
Women												
I	16	(6)	14	(5)	32	(12)	22	(8)	16	(6)	100	(37)
II	9	(6)	22	(14)	14	(9)	26	(17)	29	(19)	100	(65)
III	4	(1)	22	(6)	19	(5)	22	(6)	33	(9)	100	(27)
IV	16	(5)	15	(5)	39	(12)	16	(5)	14	(4)	100	(31)

[a]Index ranges from I (least connections) to IV (most connections).

porting no health problem; (2) those reporting one or more symptoms; (3) those reporting one or more chronic conditions; and (4) those reporting at least some disability. Men's and women's age-adjusted mortality rates in relation to the Social Network Index and the Physical Health Spectrum appear in Table 4-4. As expected, there is a considerable mortality gradient with the Physical Health Spectrum.

It is also clear that the Social Network Index predicts mortality throughout the Physical Health Spectrum. In every category of health status, both men and women with the most social contacts have lower mortality rates than those who are most isolated. The gradient from high to low in the four network categories is fairly consistent $(P \le .001)$, with only an occasional deviation, though it is least clear for women who reported having no health problem or few symptoms. These data provide further evidence that the association between social networks and mortality is not merely the reflection of underlying poor health.

SOCIAL NETWORK AND VARIOUS CAUSES OF DEATH

Another concern is that the Social Network Index may be associated with only one or two causes of death. Then the association with overall mortality could reflect these particular disease-specific relationships. In order to resolve this question, mortality rates for four separate group-causes of death were examined: (1) ischemic heart disease, (2) cerebrovascular and other circulatory disease, (3) cancer, and (4) all other causes of death—classified according to the eighth revision of the *International Classification of Diseases*.

Table 4-4. Age-adjusted mortality rates from all causes (per 100): Social Network Index and Physical Health Spectrum, men and women ages 30–69, 1965–1974

Social Network Index[a]	Physical health spectrum									
	Disability	(N)	Chronic condition	(N)	Symptom	(N)	No health problem	(N)	Total	(N)
Men										
I	—	(23)[b]	13.9	(62)	—	(29)[b]	8.1	(44)	15.6	(158)
II	28.2	(54)	9.7	(189)	14.3	(152)	8.6	(210)	12.2	(605)
III	18.0	(40)	8.8	(270)	6.0	(181)	5.6	(211)	8.6	(702)
IV	18.5	(45)	6.3	(258)	4.8	(183)	5.4	(278)	6.9	(764)
Total (N)	22.7	(162)	8.6	(779)	8.1	(545)	6.5	(743)	9.5	(2229)
Women										
I	23.0	(53)	8.3	(81)	7.0	(74)	7.7	(68)	12.1	(276)
II	12.2	(112)	8.3	(312)	2.7	(247)	4.5	(189)	7.2	(860)
III	12.8	(55)	4.2	(209)	3.1	(201)	2.8	(137)	4.9	(602)
IV	6.6	(72)	2.7	(263)	4.3	(226)	5.1	(197)	4.3	(758)
Total (N)	14.1	(292)	5.8	(865)	3.8	(748)	4.5	(591)	6.4	(2496)

[a]Index ranges from I (least connections) to IV (most connections).
[b]Rates not calculated for cells with 30 or fewer individuals.

Table 4-5 reveals that for every group-cause of death examined, isolated people had higher mortality rates than those with more social ties. Thus it appears that the Social Network Index is predictive of mortality from a wide variety of diseases. This finding lends support to the idea that social networks influence health status through a mechanism involving general resistance to disease.

Sociostructural constraints on social networks

Social networks assume forms that reflect the broad structure of society and an individual's position in the social structure (Craven and Wellman, 1973; Tilly, 1972). As societies develop from agricultural to industrialized urban forms, the emerging class systems, conflicts among different ethnic and migrating groups, and shifting populations exert pressure on individuals to structure their social relationships in certain patterns. In the midst of social change, however, people may have a difficult time maintaining social relationships or forming new ones once these are lost.

In this section we examine various sociostructural factors in relation to social networks and mortality. Previous studies had indicated that five such factors are related to both network structure and health status: (1) social class, (2) race, (3) level of urbanization, (4) geographic mobility,

Table 4-5. Age-adjusted mortality rates from selected causes (per 100): Social Network Index, men and women ages 30–69, 1965–1974

Social Network Index[a]	Cause of death					
	Ischemic heart disease	Cerebrovascular, other circulatory	Cancer	Other[b]	Total	(N)
Men						
I	5.1	2.7	2.7	4.9	15.6	(158)
II	4.3	1.2	2.6	4.1	12.3	(605)
III	4.0	0.6	0.7	2.7	8.6	(702)
IV	2.4	1.2	1.6	1.6	6.9	(764)
Total	3.6	1.1	1.8	2.9	9.5	(2229)
Women						
I	3.2	1.6	2.4	5.1	12.1	(276)
II	1.9	0.9	2.6	2.0	7.3	(860)
III	1.0	1.3	1.3	1.4	4.9	(602)
IV	1.0	0.5	1.1	1.7	4.3	(758)
Total	1.6	1.0	1.8	2.1	6.4	(2496)

[a]Index ranges from I (least connections) to IV (most connections).
[b]Other causes of death include diseases of respiratory and digestive systems, accidents, suicide.

and (5) occupational mobility. A sixth variable, utilization of preventive health services, is also included because of its potentially confounding effect, even though it is not a sociostructural variable.

One aim here is to ascertain the relationship between each of several sociostructural elements and social networks. It should be noted that the data for both come from the 1965 survey. Such cross-sectional data permit us to determine, for example, whether isolated people are likely to be in lower-class groups, to experience greater occupational and geographic mobility, or to come from urbanized areas; but they do not reveal cause and effect.

The second aim is to assess whether the Social Network Index predicted mortality independently of other social variables. Because the latter are correlated with various measures of poor health status, it is important to know whether social isolation is associated with increased mortality only because of some underlying association with race or socioeconomic status that is known to be connected with poor health.

SOCIOECONOMIC STATUS AND SOCIAL NETWORKS

Social class seems to have a pervasive influence on network structure and interaction. Poor people have less stable marriages and fewer ties to the broad community; poor older women have fewer close friends than women in the middle and upper classes. On the other hand, some evidence suggests that people in lower classes maintain strong ties to extended family members and non-kin that provide a solid basis for support. In her ethnographic study of poor black women living in a rural community, Stack (1974), concludes:

Black families in the flats and the non-kin they regard as kin have evolved patterns of co-residence, kinship-based exchange networks linking multiple domestic units, elastic household boundaries, life-long bonds of three generation households, and social controls against the formation of marriages that could endanger the network of kin.

Furthermore, social class is consistently associated with a wide variety of health outcomes. People in the lower social classes have higher morbidity and mortality rates from almost all causes and are also more inclined to certain behaviors that induce poor health, such as smoking and being overweight (Syme and Berkman, 1976). It is possible that social networks predict mortality because of their underlying association with social class or, conversely, that social class is associated with health because of its relationship to networks. Thus the vast amount of evidence relating social class to network structures and health demands that the interaction among these three variables be examined in some depth.

Measures of income and educational level included in the 1965 HPL survey were used to develop an index of socioeconomic status. Each of the two measures, income level and educational level, was then used to construct five categories approximating a normal curve, with the middle category containing about a third of the sample, the two surrounding groups about 20 percent each, and the two extreme categories about 15 percent each. Combining income and education categories then yielded five new groups.

Figure 4-4 reveals a strong positive association between socioeconomic status and extent of social contacts. Among both men and women, the lower the social class the greater the social isolation. The gradient is particularly striking among women 30–59 years of age. In that group between 60 and 70% of lower-class women but only 25% of upper-class women score low on the Social Network Index. Generally, social class is highly correlated with the extent of social contacts as measured by the index.

Analysis of the four separate components of the Social Network Index —marital status, close friends and relatives, church groups, and nonchurch groups—revealed that people of low socioeconomic level ranked lower than those in the upper classes on three components of the index. Only with respect to close friends and relatives do lower-class men and women compare favorably with those in the upper classes. The relative extensiveness of lower-class persons' contacts with friends and extended family, particularly among men, has been documented by ethnographers such as Stack (1974), Whyte (1965), Liebow (1967), and Gans (1962). These contacts have been described as major sources of support in the face of other considerable social, economic, and personal losses. Having close friends and relatives may thus be an important resource for poor people who lack other kinds of social connections.

In order to examine the relationship among socioeconomic groups, social networks, and mortality, the Social Network Index was collapsed from four categories to two, because of small numbers of deaths in some cells.

Table 4-6 shows age-adjusted mortality rates among persons 30–69 years of age in relation to the Social Network and socioeconomic indices. In all five social class categories both men and women with few social contacts had higher mortality rates than those with many connections ($P \leq .001$). These data support the conclusion that the Social Network Index predicts mortality independently of socioeconomic status.

The findings presented in this chapter indicate that an individual's social network may be partly determined by socioeconomic level. In his essay on culture and poverty, however, Valentine (1968) has emphasized

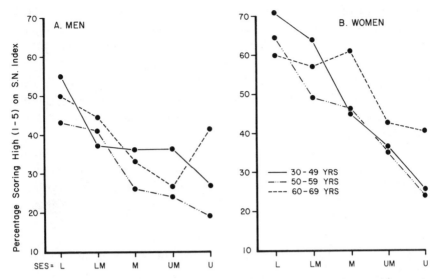

Fig. 4-4. Percentage scoring high on Social Network (S.N.) Index among five socioeconomic status (SES) groups, age- and sex-specific rates, 1965.

that although the poor possess some distinct subcultural patterns, they are still a heterogeneous population with variable and adaptive subcultures. The HPL data also suggest that the socioeconomic classes are not homogeneous with regard to network form. For example, although they were a minority, some lower-class men and women had very adequate social connections. Thus although the form of networks may reflect class position to a certain extent, clearly other factors also play a role in shaping network structure.

The possibility that other kinds of social connections, not tapped by the 1965 survey, are available to people in the lower classes and provide support equivalent to the Social Network Index used here should be explored in future work. However, the fact that the index, as simply constructed as it is, does predict mortality across all social classes suggests that these measures are applicable to people in different socioeconomic groups.

GEOGRAPHIC MOBILITY

Geographic mobility adversely affects an individual's ability to maintain social contacts, and such mobility has also been reported to have certain deleterious health consequences. Thus it is possible that the association between social isolation and mortality risk is a result of some underlying relationship among networks, geographic mobility, and mortality. To

Table 4-6. Age-adjusted mortality rates from all causes (per 100): Social Network Index and socioeconomic status, men and women ages 30–69, 1965–1974

Social Network Index[a]	Socioeconomic status											
	Lower	(N)	Lower middle	(N)	Middle	(N)	Upper middle	(N)	Upper	(N)	Total	(N)
Men												
I and II	11.8	(86)	12.7	(110)	16.6	(243)	11.7	(242)	7.3	(67)	13.1	(748)
III and IV	8.0	(89)	11.1	(168)	6.3	(501)	8.1	(498)	4.2	(192)	7.5	(1448)
Total (N)	9.9	(175)	11.7	(278)	9.5	(744)	9.1	(740)	5.2	(259)	9.4	(2196)
Women												
I and II	9.9	(121)	7.3	(209)	8.2	(431)	6.8	(302)	5.7	(40)	8.0	(1103)
III and IV	7.3	(69)	1.1	(151)	4.9	(487)	4.1	(514)	5.2	(123)	4.4	(1344)
Total (N)	8.8	(190)	4.6	(360)	6.6	(918)	5.2	(816)	5.4	(163)	6.1	(2447)

[a]Index ranges from I (least connections) to IV (most connections).

answer this question from the HPL data, age-adjusted mortality rates were examined within a matrix of levels of geographic mobility and social contact.

Geographic mobility was measured by responses to a single question on the 1965 questionnaire: "During the last 5 years, how many addresses have you lived at? (Count the address you are living at now.)" Respondents to this item were divided into three categories: (1) those living at one address, (2) those living at two addresses, and (3) those living at three or more addresses in the last 5 years.

Those who moved two or more times in the 5 years preceding the 1965 survey were more likely to die in the follow-up period than those who did not move or moved only once. An association between social isolation and mobility was found that is especially strong for older men, and for younger and middle-aged women. As seen in Table 4-7, the Social Network Index continues to predict mortality independently of geographic mobility. In each category of geographic mobility with only minor deviations, the social network/mortality gradient is observed. The relationship between networks and mortality persists for both men and women when controlling for both age and geographic mobility ($P \leq .001$). However, the relationship between mobility and mortality is almost obscured when controlling for level of social contact. Whether this finding reflects the ability of social connections to reduce the impact of numerous moves on mortality, or is due to a weak association between geographic mobility

Table 4-7. Age-adjusted mortality rates from all causes (per 100): Social Network Index and geographic mobility, men and women ages 30–69, 1965–1974

Social Network Index[a]	Number of addresses in last 5 years							
	One	(N)	Two	(N)	Three or more	(N)	Total	(N)
Men								
I	15.2	(62)	23.5	(39)	13.7	(51)	16.6	(152)
II	11.3	(260)	10.4	(151)	15.8	(169)	11.9	(580)
III	8.6	(349)	6.7	(182)	10.6	(160)	8.5	(691)
IV	6.1	(417)	8.1	(193)	8.2	(136)	6.9	(746)
Total (N)	8.7	(1088)	9.4	(565)	12.0	(516)	9.4	(2169)
Women								
I	7.9	(104)	12.2	(78)	19.2	(79)	11.7	(261)
II	7.2	(407)	5.8	(218)	7.9	(201)	7.0	(826)
III	5.2	(332)	4.1	(155)	4.1	(100)	4.8	(587)
IV	4.4	(470)	4.5	(175)	3.0	(104)	4.2	(749)
Total (N)	5.8	(1313)	6.0	(626)	8.3	(484)	6.2	(2423)

[a]Index ranges from I (least connections) to IV (most connections).

and mortality is uncertain. In either case, this analysis suggests that whereas social isolation is associated with geographic mobility, the relationship between social isolation and mortality risk cannot be attributed to the geographic mobility of those who lack many social ties.

OCCUPATIONAL MOBILITY

Occupational mobility could also possibly influence both health status and social networks. In the present analysis only those men and women who were employed in the last 10 years were included; the total sample size was thus significantly reduced because less than half the women worked outside the home during the 10 years before the survey. Occupational mobility was measured by an individual's response to the question: "During the past 10 years, how many different companies have you worked for?" Responses were categorized as follows: (1) those working for one company, (2) those working for two companies, and (3) those working for three or more companies in the past 10 years. It should be noted that this item does not measure upward or downward occupational mobility, advancements, or demotions, but only job changes from one company to another.

Table 4-8 shows age-adjusted mortality rates for the Social Network Index according to numbers of job changes in the 10 years preceding the

Table 4-8. Age-adjusted mortality rates from all causes (per 100): Social Network Index and occupational mobility, men and women ages 30–69, 1965–1974

Social Network Index[a]	Number of job changes in last 10 years[b]							
	One	(N)	Two	(N)	Three or more	(N)	Total	(N)
Men								
I	11.5	(54)	—	(24)[c]	7.8	(36)	9.6	(114)
II	10.6	(260)	9.4	(111)	10.2	(164)	10.3	(535)
III	6.8	(318)	9.8	(153)	5.8	(180)	7.2	(651)
IV	5.6	(350)	4.5	(188)	6.6	(165)	5.5	(703)
Total (N)	7.6	(982)	7.4	(476)	7.6	(545)	7.5	(2003)
Women								
I	10.4	(55)	0.0	(35)	18.9	(33)	9.3	(123)
II	5.3	(198)	1.9	(108)	5.9	(103)	4.7	(409)
III	2.8	(137)	3.3	(64)	3.7	(58)	3.1	(259)
IV	3.4	(165)	4.2	(87)	2.4	(48)	3.4	(300)
Total (N)	4.6	(555)	2.7	(294)	6.4	(242)	4.5	(1091)

[a]Index ranges from I (least connections) to IV (most connections).
[b]Includes only those men and women employed in last 10 years.
[c]Rates not calculated for cells with 30 or fewer individuals.

1965 survey. Only among women who worked for three or more companies was there any increase in mortality risk associated with occupational mobility. Both men and women who have worked for three companies or more tended to lack social ties, compared with those who worked for only one or two companies.

When controlling for occupational mobility the Social Network Index continues to predict mortality, although within some categories of job change the network/mortality gradient becomes unclear. Adjusted for both age and occupational mobility, the association between social networks and mortality is statistically significant for both men ($P \leq .01$) and women ($P \leq .05$). Thus the Social Network Index continues to predict mortality independently of one measure of occupational mobility—the number of companies a person has worked for over the past 10 years.

LEVEL OF URBANIZATION

City life may also influence an individual's ability to maintain enduring and effective social connections. Much of the literature concerning social networks has in fact focused on changes that occur when individuals migrate into urban areas, or as the areas in which they live become urbanized. It has also been suggested that urbanization itself adversely affects health status, although the evidence supporting this hypothesis is questionable.

Because Alameda County is a relatively urbanized county with few truly rural areas, it is difficult to test hypotheses about urbanization with the HPL data. However, it is possible to compare areas within the county that are relatively rural with areas that are clearly urban. For that purpose, Alameda County was divided into three areas based on characteristics of townships and census tracts: (1) rural parts, (2) urban nonpoverty areas, and (3) urban poverty areas. It seemed important to distinguish between urban poverty and nonpoverty areas because otherwise some economic characteristics of poverty areas might mistakenly be attributed to "urban life-style."

Eden, Livermore, and Washington townships—sparsely populated in 1965 and characterized by family-owned farms and orchards with mostly single-family dwellings—comprised the rural part of the county.

Oakland, the major metropolis of Alameda County, identified one area of the city for a federal antipoverty program. It consisted of contiguous census tracts with 1960 male unemployment rates of 9 percent or higher. As of 1965, about one-third of the residents of Oakland lived in this area, including the majority of the city's black population. Although it was generally conceded that the poverty area was depressed and included most of the city's poor people, most of the poverty area residents had incomes above the poverty level. Using the same criterion as in Oakland, Berkeley poverty areas were determined. The urban poverty areas for the study consisted of these parts of Oakland and Berkeley.

The remaining sections of Oakland and Berkeley and the city of Alameda comprised the urban nonpoverty area. Although the data are not shown here, the Social Network Index and level of urbanization were not consistently associated. Both men and women under the age of 60 living in rural areas had stronger social networks than those living in urban non-poverty or poverty areas. On the other hand, older rural women had the weakest social ties of any group. Thus at younger ages rural people seem to have stronger social ties, but at older ages urban dwellers, especially those living in nonpoverty areas, tend to have stronger social networks.

Table 4-9 displays age-adjusted mortality rates according to the Social Network Index and level of urbanization. Persons living in urban poverty areas had a particularly high mortality risk. Within each level of urbanization, however, the Social Network Index continues to predict mortality consistently. Thus social isolation was associated with mortality independently of the level of urbanization. Adjusting for both age and level of urbanization, the association between isolation and increased mortality risk remains statistically significant for both men and women ($P \leq .001$).

Table 4-9. Age-adjusted mortality rates from all causes (per 100): Social Network Index and level of urbanization, men and women ages 30–69, 1965–1974

Social Network Index[a]	Level of urbanization							
	Urban (poverty)	(N)	Urban (nonpoverty)	(N)	Rural	(N)	Total	(N)
Men								
I	20.5	(45)	12.1	(71)	15.9	(42)	15.6	(158)
II	14.7	(115)	12.8	(271)	10.0	(219)	12.3	(605)
III	10.0	(79)	8.9	(273)	7.8	(350)	8.6	(702)
IV	8.4	(111)	7.8	(286)	5.2	(367)	6.9	(764)
Total (N)	12.2	(350)	9.9	(901)	7.7	(978)	9.5	(2229)
Women								
I	16.6	(68)	10.8	(112)	10.5	(96)	12.1	(276)
II	11.5	(163)	6.1	(368)	6.0	(329)	7.3	(860)
III	7.2	(67)	5.0	(257)	3.8	(278)	4.9	(602)
IV	6.9	(119)	4.4	(314)	2.7	(325)	4.3	(758)
Total (N)	10.4	(417)	5.9	(1051)	5.1	(1028)	6.4	(2496)

[a]Index ranges from I (least connections) to IV (most connections).

The urban/rural gradient in mortality within each category of the Social Network Index indicates that urbanization is associated with an increase in mortality risk independently of the extent to which people maintain social ties.

RACE

None of the analyses described thus far have taken into account possible differences among racial groups with respect to either network patterns or health. In order to examine racial and ethnic patterns of social networks and how these might be related to mortality, mortality rates were calculated along the Social Network Index for three different racial and/or ethnic groups: whites, blacks, and all others (Mexican, Japanese, and Chinese Americans, and all other nonwhites). For every age and sex group, except women 60–69, whites scored higher on the Social Network Index than either blacks or all others. Whites were more likely to belong to nonchurch groups and to be married, but blacks were more likely to be church members and also showed a tendency to have more contacts with friends and relatives.

Table 4-10 shows age-adjusted mortality rates according to the Social Network Index for the three different racial and ethnic groups. Although an association exists between networks and racial groups, the Social Net-

Table 4-10. Age-adjusted mortality rates from all causes (per 100): Social Network Index and race, men and women ages 30–69, 1965–1974

Social Network Index[a]	Race							
	White	(N)	Black	(N)	Other	(N)	Total	(N)
Men								
I	13.7	(109)	—	(29)[b]	—	(20)[b]	15.6	(158)
II	12.7	(468)	11.6	(81)	9.8	(56)	12.3	(605)
III	8.2	(592)	10.3	(64)	8.9	(46)	8.6	(702)
IV	6.5	(618)	9.1	(108)	7.1	(36)	6.9	(762)
Total (N)	9.2	(1787)	11.2	(282)	10.2	(158)	9.5	(2227)
Women								
I	13.0	(192)	10.3	(47)	8.4	(37)	12.1	(276)
II	6.2	(674)	13.1	(120)	8.3	(66)	7.3	(860)
III	4.6	(501)	7.6	(65)	3.3	(34)	4.9	(600)
IV	3.5	(606)	8.9	(127)	—	(24)[b]	4.3	(757)
Total (N)	5.8	(1973)	10.3	(359)	6.0	(161)	6.4	(2493)

[a]Index ranges from I (least connections) to IV (most connections).
[b]Rates not calculated for cells with 30 or fewer individuals.

work Index continues to predict mortality independently of racial status, with statistical significance ($P \leq .001$ for both men and women).

It is also clear from these data that mortality is associated with racial status. Among both men and women, blacks have higher mortality rates than whites and other racial and ethnic groups. These differences are generally, though not consistently, observable within each category of the Social Network Index. This suggests that though varying network structure among different races may account for some of the mortality difference, other factors also appear to influence the racial gradient of mortality observed in these data.

PREVENTIVE HEALTH SERVICES

Another possibility is that the relationship between social networks and mortality, which is not explained by any of the social factors considered thus far, could be explained by differential use of medical services by people with few social resources. In order to examine this issue, an index of preventive health service utilization was developed based on two questions: (1) "Have you had a dental checkup in the past year, even though you felt well?" and (2) "Have you had a medical checkup in the past year, even though you felt well?" Respondents who answered yes to both were scored high; the low group consisted of respondents who had neither a dental nor a medical checkup; moderate scorers were those who had one or the other.

Age-adjusted mortality rates for the Social Network Index and the index of preventive utilization of health services appear in Table 4-11. Men and women who used preventive health services the most experienced somewhat lower mortality rates than those who reported no or moderate use of the specified services. The social network gradient in mortality persists throughout the preventive health care categories ($P \leq .005$). Although this index is probably not a very sensitive measure of preventive health services, variations in mortality observed among people with different extents of social connections cannot be explained by an obvious, gross difference in use of preventive health services.

Psychological variables

Psychological states, it is often suggested, may either mediate the relationship between social networks and mortality, or affect people's networks directly. According to the first hypothesis, people without social ties become lonely, depressed, or alienated, and some such psychological state induces illness. According to the second hypothesis, people who are

Table 4-11. Age-adjusted mortality rates from all causes (per 100): Social Network Index and level of preventive care, men and women ages 30–69, 1965–1974

Social Network Index[a]	Level of preventive health care							
	Low	(N)	Medium	(N)	High	(N)	Total	(N)
Men								
I	15.4	(49)	9.7	(48)	—	(29)[b]	14.2	(126)
II	11.4	(162)	9.8	(203)	9.2	(118)	10.2	(483)
III	7.8	(180)	6.5	(236)	4.5	(170)	6.1	(586)
IV	5.8	(181)	5.6	(241)	6.1	(197)	5.8	(619)
Total (N)	8.6	(572)	7.8	(728)	6.9	(514)	7.7	(1814)
Women								
I	6.8	(66)	11.4	(78)	8.4	(50)	8.8	(194)
II	8.4	(171)	5.4	(241)	5.4	(236)	6.1	(648)
III	2.7	(115)	6.7	(199)	4.0	(184)	4.7	(498)
IV	3.6	(117)	3.5	(238)	3.6	(253)	3.6	(608)
Total (N)	5.6	(469)	5.6	(756)	4.6	(723)	5.2	(1948)

[a]Index ranges from I (least connections) to IV (most connections).
[b]Rates not calculated for cells with 30 or fewer individuals.

mentally disturbed, depressed, or asocial find it difficult to maintain social ties because of their psychological makeup. In this case, social isolation would be a situational response to some psychological characteristic.

In order to explore these issues, the psychological characteristics ascertained in the 1965 survey were subjected to a factor analysis that yielded seven distinct and unidimensional factors. This analysis was conducted because some of the originally developed indices were of unknown validity. Precise descriptions of items are given in the Appendix.

The cross-sectional associations between the psychological factors and social networks are generally modest. The coefficients from a Pearson product-moment correlation, correcting for age, are statistically significant but small (Table 4-12). This indicates that the Social Network Index measures something distinct from the psychological factors studied. Each of the seven psychological factors and their relationships to mortality and social networks will be discussed only briefly here. More data on these relationships are given in the Appendix.

The first factor was composed of six items from an index of neurotic traits and a seventh from an anomy scale (McCloskey and Scharr, 1965). Typical items were as follows: "I am easily sidetracked." "I have a hard time making up my mind." "I'm not sure what I really want most of the time." People who score high on the index might be described as un-

Table 4-12. Partial coefficients, controlling for age, Social Network Index, and psychological factors, men and women ages 30–69, 1965

Factor	Coefficient	Statistical significance (P)
Men		
1. Personal uncertainty	−.12	.001
2. Anomy	−.05	.008
3. Life satisfaction	.20	.001
4. Social insecurity	−.12	.001
5. Perfectionism	−.05	.009
6. Negative feelings	−.13	.001
7. Isolation/depression	−.23	.001
Women		
1. Personal uncertainty	−.10	.001
2. Anomy	−.08	.001
3. Life satisfaction	.17	.001
4. Social insecurity	−.16	.001
5. Perfectionism	−.09	.001
6. Negative feelings	−.19	.001
7. Isolation/depression	−.27	.001

certain or unsure. They appear to lack some kind of directedness, immobilizing them from making decisions. The Social Network Index continues to predict mortality independently of this factor, but personal uncertainty also exerts a modest influence on mortality independently of social networks (see Appendix).

The second factor includes seven of the original nine items in the anomy scale developed by McCloskey and Scharr (1965). They reflect an individual's sense of normlessness in the world around him, for example: "With everything in a state of disorder, it's hard for a person to know where he stands." "People were better off in the old days when everyone knew just how he was expected to act." "What is lacking in the world today is the old kind of friendship that lasted for a lifetime." This factor is not significantly associated with mortality and fails to affect the network/mortality gradient. Therefore, anomy measured in this way neither enhances nor diminishes the relationship between reported social isolation and risk of death (see Appendix).

Among the seven psychological factors studied here the most important in predicting mortality risk consists of all six positive-feeling items from Bradburn and Caplovitz (1965), and three questions concerning satisfaction in major life roles. The following items were typical: "How often do you feel on top of the world?" "How happy are you these days?" and

"Have your marriage, kids, and job turned out as you expected and been satisfying?" Table 4-13 shows the age-adjusted mortality rates for the Social Network Index and this third factor, which is called life satisfaction. The relative risk for this factor alone approaches 2 for men and 3 for women. As may be seen, the Social Network Index predicts mortality independently of this expression of life satisfaction; the latter also predicts mortality independently of the extent of social networks. Moreover, there is a good deal of interaction between the two variables; in fact, they approach an additive effect. People who are most isolated and also score lowest on the life satisfaction scale are approximately 4.5 times more likely to die than people with many social connections who also report many life satisfactions. These findings suggest that both the objective circumstances of social life and subjectively evaluated life satisfaction play a role in determining health status. In other words, social and psychological phenomena interact to produce biologic consequences.

Most of the items in the fourth factor come from an index of *ego resiliency* developed by Block (1965), who defined it as "resourcefulness, adaptability, and engagement in the world." Reflecting feelings of social threat and insecurity, typical examples are: "It's hard for me to start a conversation with strangers," "I feel nervous if I have to meet a lot of people," "I often feel awkward and out of place," and "I feel left out of a group even if they are friends of mine." Although these items suggest difficulty in maintaining social contacts, the factor is only weakly correlated with the Social Network Index and is unrelated to mortality. This psychological dimension does not decrease the power of the Social Network Index to predict mortality (see Appendix).

The fifth factor consists of items measuring perfectionism, for example: "I'm never quite satisfied with what I do," and "Even when other people praise my work, I'm still dissatisfied." It shows no relationship to either mortality or social networks, and the Social Network Index continues to predict mortality independently of psychological perfectionism (see Appendix).

Items in the sixth factor come almost entirely from the five negative-feeling statements of the Bradburn-Caplovitz index: "How often do you feel depressed or very unhappy, . . . very lonely or remote from others, . . . vaguely uneasy about something without knowing why, . . . bored, . . . restless?" It shows a moderate but consistent association with mortality. Both men and women with strong negative feelings experienced higher mortality rates than persons with weaker feelings of that sort. Once again, however, the mortality gradient with social networks is not attributable to negative feelings (see Appendix).

Table 4-13. Age-adjusted mortality rates from all causes (per 100): Social Network Index and life satisfaction, men and women ages 30–69, 1965–1974

Social Network Index[a]	Level of life satisfaction							
	Low	(N)	Medium	(N)	High	(N)	Total	(N)
Men								
I	20.6	(80)	6.6	(49)	17.6	(24)	15.9	(153)
II	14.0	(224)	12.2	(252)	7.3	(121)	12.2	(597)
III	9.5	(215)	8.1	(294)	9.2	(192)	8.5	(701)
IV	9.4	(163)	6.8	(336)	4.6	(262)	6.8	(761)
Total (N)	12.8	(682)	8.4	(931)	7.1	(599)	9.3	(2212)
Women								
I	15.8	(138)	8.5	(83)	3.8	(48)	11.7	(269)
II	9.8	(350)	6.2	(314)	3.9	(189)	8.6	(853)
III	6.7	(190)	5.3	(247)	1.3	(164)	4.9	(601)
IV	6.8	(214)	2.6	(279)	3.4	(262)	4.1	(755)
Total (N)	9.4	(892)	5.0	(923)	3.3	(663)	6.3	(2478)

[a]Index ranges from I (least connections) to IV (most connections).

The final cluster of items represents feelings of isolation and depression, for example: "I tend to keep people at a distance." "It's hard for me to feel close to others." "I find it easy to drop or break with a friend." "It often seems that my life has no meaning." Of all the seven psychological factors considered, this one is the most highly correlated with Social Network Index. This is not surprising because both measure dimensions of isolation. The seventh factor measures a psychological attitude that discourages contacts with others, typified by the item: "I tend to keep people at a distance." The Social Network Index, on the other hand, measures actual contacts without attention to attitudes or feelings about social relationships. If there is a psychological characteristic that determines the extent of one's social network, however, this factor seems a likely candidate. Analyzing that characteristic, then, might be considered the best way of testing, in this data set, whether some psychological factor influences the formation of social networks and underlies the association between networks and mortality.

People who score high on the isolation/depression index tend to have slightly higher mortality rates than those in the middle and lower range of feeling isolated and depressed. For neither men nor women, however, did the age-adjusted differences in mortality reach statistical significance. This modest association of isolation/depression with mortality is surprising because that psychological factor is highly correlated with the Social

Network Index. Evidently, the Social Network Index's ability to predict mortality does not result from an underlying association between this psychological factor and mortality risk (Table 4-14).

The data thus do not support the hypothesis that some psychological factors influence social network formation and are responsible for the mortality gradient observed among people with varying degrees of social connection.

Analysis of psychological variables and interactions among them has obviously been limited by the kinds of questions asked in the 1965 survey. It might be argued that the important psychological items affecting health were simply not asked. This analysis would then not truly indicate whether psychological states or traits predict mortality. Support for the notion that psychological characteristics may play some role in predicting disease may be found in work by Rosenman et al. (1976) and Jenkins et al. (1974), revealing that the type A behavior pattern is associated with coronary heart disease; by Schmale and Iker (1966), LeShan (1966), and Bahnson and Bahnson (1966), suggesting that "hopelessness" or having a "lack of emotional outlets" and "denial" may promote the development of cancer; and by Lazarus and his colleagues (1962), indicating that coping and appraisal processes may be involved in stress responses. These psychological characteristics or processes are not represented by the factors developed from the HPL data.

Table 4-14. Age-adjusted mortality rates from all causes (per 100): Social Network Index and isolation/depression, men and women ages 30–69, 1965–1974

Social Network Index[a]	Level of isolation/depression							
	High	(N)	Medium	(N)	Low	(N)	Total	(N)
Men								
I	14.0	(67)	16.1	(53)	15.1	(34)	14.9	(154)
II	14.2	(223)	7.5	(224)	12.4	(150)	12.0	(597)
III	10.5	(148)	7.5	(311)	8.9	(237)	9.4	(696)
IV	7.2	(112)	6.9	(323)	6.6	(326)	6.9	(761)
Total (N)	11.9	(550)	8.4	(911)	8.8	(747)	9.4	(2208)
Women								
I	11.2	(106)	12.8	(114)	9.8	(50)	11.7	(270)
II	9.3	(259)	6.2	(359)	6.3	(236)	7.0	(854)
III	1.6	(122)	6.7	(238)	4.7	(240)	4.9	(600)
IV	7.1	(82)	3.2	(288)	4.5	(384)	4.2	(754)
Total (N)	7.8	(569)	5.4	(999)	5.4	(910)	6.3	(2478)

[a]Index ranges from I (least connections) to IV (most connections).

To conclude, the findings do indicate that (1) the relationship between the Social Network Index and mortality does not result from any underlying psychological phenomena examined, and (2) social network and self-reported life satisfaction together form a powerful predictor of mortality, stronger than either alone.

Summary and discussion

The preceding analyses have shown the risk of mortality to be associated with four types of social relationships: (1) marriage, (2) contacts with close friends and relatives, (3) church membership, and (4) associations with nonchurch groups. In each instance, people with such social relationships had lower mortality rates than people without them. The more intimate ties of marriage and contact with close friends and relatives were stronger predictors than were church and nonchurch group membership.

To assess the cumulative effects of these social relationships, a Social Network Index was developed from the data on these four types of contact. When the sample was stratified according to type and degree of affiliation, the most isolated group of men had an age-adjusted mortality rate 2.3 times higher than men with the strongest social connections; among women who were most isolated, the rate was 2.8 times higher than among women with the strongest social connections. With one minor exception, for every age group examined, and for both sexes, people with the strongest social network had the lowest mortality rates and people with the weakest social network had the highest rates. The relative risks ranged from just under 2 to more than 4.5.

The association between the Social Network Index and mortality was independent of physical health at the time of the survey, year of death, socioeconomic status, race and other social and demographic factors, utilization of preventive health services, and many psychological factors.

A number of different social relationships can apparently affect placement in a particular risk category. For instance, people who were not married but had many close friends and relatives had mortality rates equal to those who were married but who had few contacts with close friends and relatives. Similarly, it did not seem important whether contacts were among close friends or among relatives; only the absence of both was related to increased risk of death during the follow-up period. Tradeoffs such as these apparently helped about 60 percent of the sample, through one kind of contact or another, to maintain a relatively low mortality risk. Only in the presence of severe social disconnection, when individuals failed generally to have social links, did mortality rates rise sharply.

Limitations of mortality data

Two limitations involved in the use of mortality as an end point have implications for the conclusions that can be drawn from these results. First, there is the possibility that people who died during the 9-year follow-up period were ill at the time of the initial survey. The association between physical health status, as determined at the baseline survey, and subsequent mortality supports this suspicion. It is therefore conceivable that the relationship found between networks and mortality existed because isolated people were ill at the time of the survey and were physically unable to maintain extended contacts. This is a serious issue and one that was explored in some depth. The results presented, however, do not support this possible explanation. While controlling for health status at the time of the baseline survey, the Social Network Index continued to predict mortality. In an analysis of year of death, it was shown that the percentage of deaths occurring in the first years following the survey among isolated people is similar to the respective percentage of deaths among those with many social contacts. If these two analyses involved valid and accurate indicators of illness status at the time of the survey, it does not appear likely that the relationship between networks and mortality is merely a reflection of underlying poor health. On the other hand, if these measures are not valid and accurate indices of health status in 1965, this issue remains unresolved.

The second limitation of mortality data is likewise related to the association between mortality and morbidity. Throughout this report, the implication has been that social factors influence susceptibility to disease, that is, disease incidence. In fact, from studies involving mortality data alone, it cannot be ascertained whether the risk factors influence disease incidence or instead "survival time" between the onset or diagnosis of disease and death. It should be noted that in either case host resistance may be the mechanism involved. An analysis in Chapter 6 of the relationship between social networks and subsequent health status will help to resolve some of these issues.

The functions of social networks

Although the findings summarized above and presented in detail earlier confirm the relationship between mortality and social relationships and activities, they raise many issues that cannot be directly answered by further analyses of these data. For instance, one can only speculate why social networks are related to health status or what the biologic mechanisms are that lead from social disconnection to disease and death.

In order to ascertain what it is about social networks that may be critical to the maintenance of health, it is necessary to have some understanding of the functions of social and community ties. Social network analysis generally draws on an exchange model of social relations in which interpersonal relations are conceptualized as exchanges where the content ranges from material goods, to services, to emotional support. In a review of the relationship between social supports and health, Kaplan, Cassel, and Gore (1977) summarized the three main functions of social contacts as providing tangible support, appraisal support, and emotional support.

1. People appear to need social and community ties to fulfill some very practical, tangible needs. For instance, social resources are needed to borrow money or goods, to obtain help when one is ill, or for such tasks as shopping, finding jobs, and locating and acquiring the services of doctors, lawyers, and community officials. Occasionally, people need help with transportation, housecleaning, baby-sitting, and other kinds of caretaking. People without appropriate social ties may suffer from the consequences of not having these needs fulfilled. They may have inadequate medical care or legal advice, they may find it difficult to find a job, or to go shopping or get around town, and they may be overloaded from work or household tasks with no one to relieve them. Undoubtedly, different people have varying needs depending on personal and social circumstances; yet it is likely that from time to time everyone has certain material or instrumental needs that are most effectively fulfilled by social contacts.

2. The appraisal function of social support is defined by Kaplan et al. (1977) as "help in defining role expectations." The opportunity to evaluate social situations and decide on appropriate reactions appears to be in part provided by interactions among social contacts. An example of such an appraisal function is provided by Schacter (1959), who found that when people were exposed to ambiguous situations, they had an increased desire for affiliation. He thought that this increased desire to be with people could be attributed to the need to appraise the situation and to determine the "appropriate and proper reaction."

3. Emotional needs that may be gratified through social contacts are difficult to define. However, many sociologists, psychologists, and psychiatrists agree that people have emotional needs for intimacy, a sense of belongingness and integration in society, and a need for love, affection, and nurturance. Recently, Antonovsky (1979) has proposed that a "sense of coherence" provided by situations in which people are surrounded by strong social networks, religious faith, and other environments may be a central factor in the maintenance of health. This sense of coherence is defined as the global orientation that expresses the extent to which one

has a pervasive, enduring though dynamic feeling of confidence that one's external and internal environments are predictable and that there is a high probability that things will work out as well as can reasonably be expected. These emotional needs appear to be necessary from early childhood through old age, although they may vary by stage of life and by the actors capable of fulfilling these needs.

The distinction between social networks and social support has often been blurred by investigators who use the terms interchangeably. Research approaches focusing on networks characterize the kinds of ties people have to one another. Social support approaches emphasize the nature of support individuals have. Although the two are clearly wed to one another, they are not synonymous. Indeed the most interesting question in the field may be how the structure of social networks affects the availability of support. Wellman has succinctly stated the case for distinguishing the two factors:

When we declare ahead of time that a set of ties constitutes a support system we assume in advance precisely that which we want to leave open for study. In order to study the situations under which individuals do get support, we must allow for the possibility that many of their ties are not necessarily supportive. (Wellman, 1981, p. 172)

In the present study, virtually no questions relating to social support were included in the survey. Clearly, attempts should be made in the future, to characterize an individual's social network, the kind of support received from the network, who supplies the support, and under what conditions mutually supportive situations are maintained. In this way, we will come closer to understanding precisely the dimensions of social networks that are important to health.

*Plausible biologic pathways leading
from social disconnection to disease*

The mechanisms by which conditions in the social environment might influence health status in human populations are a relatively unexplored area. In a search for such pathways, it is important to keep in mind that social conditions—networks in particular—seem to be associated with a wide range of health outcomes rather than any single disease entity. This indicates that either there are several pathways leading from social circumstances to illness, such circumstances lead to compromised resistance to disease in general, or both. As Cassel (1976), a proponent of the latter hypothesis, suggests, it may also be that there are several clusters of diseases associated with different psychosocial situations.

If we take the view that there are likely to be multiple biologic pathways, several possibilities can be outlined: (1) behavioral processes whereby people living in certain social and cultural circumstances maintain health practices that are either beneficial (e.g., physical activity) or harmful (e.g., cigarette smoking) to their health; (2) psychological processes whereby people respond to circumstances by becoming depressed or changing their coping and appraisal processes; (3) direct physiological effects both on known biologic risk factors (e.g., blood pressure, serum cholesterol) and on unidentified processes that are directly altered by exposure to certain environmental circumstances. In the exploration of this chain leading from environmental conditions to health outcomes, we must also recognize that the direction of causality can be reversed. It is possible, for instance, that psychological states such as depression could influence social conditions. Studies in which these variables are being investigated will be most useful if the temporal order of events can be identified. It is also likely that characteristics of the person and the environment in combination will ultimately be the best predictors of disease risk.

Behavioral factors including health practices, preventive utilization of health services, and compliance with treatment regimens are obvious candidates as links between socioenvironmental conditions and disease consequences; however, the HPL data indicate that health practices are capable of explaining only a small part of the association between social isolation and increased morbidity and mortality risk. It is important to remember, however, that the HPL association between social disconnection and high-risk health practices was cross-sectional. In addition, the possibility that social networks provide instrumental aid to individuals (taking care of and feeding ill people, providing access to good medical care, helping individuals follow therapeutic regimens) was not evaluated.

Psychological factors such as depression or coping processes also seem likely candidates as mediators between environmental conditions and illness responses, and there is some literature to support this view. Of particular interest is the work of Seligman (1975), Rotter (1966), and others on feelings of internal and external control and learned helplessness, and a review of coping mechanisms and social circumstances by Satariano and Syme (1981). These investigators have hypothesized that when individuals are habitually confronted with situations in which their responses are or appear to be ineffective, they ultimately come to conclude that events in general are uncontrollable and that they are powerless to effect a particular outcome. Seligman (1975) suggests that such feelings are related to depression and perhaps to other health problems. Psychological responses may also predispose an individual to suicide or risk-taking that could result in accidents. Engel and Schmale (1972) and Antonovsky (1979) underline the importance to health maintenance of "giving up" as opposed to having a sense of control or "coherence." There is as yet little strong evidence to support these positions by predicting physical health status or linking socioenvironmental processes to health outcomes in human populations. However, it is interesting to note their similarity with Cassel's characterization (1976) of stressful social situations as ones in which "the actor is not receiving adequate evidence (feedback) that his actions are leading to anticipated consequences." Social isolation might well be the prime example of such a situation.

Whereas this suggests that the role social factors play in disease causation does not arise from circumstances themselves, but from the way they are subjectively perceived and mediated, it is also possible that there may be a pathway leading directly from social circumstances to physiological changes in the body that increase either general or specific disease susceptibility. The finding in the HPL study that no psychological factors developed from items on the 1965 survey mediated between social isolation and mortality risk supports this view, although none of the factors was developed to measure the psychological dimensions just described.

Guided by the stress theory of disease originally formulated by Cannon (1935), Selye (1956), and Wolff (1953), Cassel (1976) described a pathway by which social factors could increase susceptibility to disease in general. According to this hypothesis, psychosocial factors influence physiological reactions by acting as signs and symbols of danger. In experimental studies such symbolic threats have been found to elicit reactions not very different from those provoked by the direct threat. According to Dubos (1965) and Cannon (1935), the balance between the organism and various disease agents is maintained by the neuroendocrine system. In Cassel's view signs and symbols exert their influence by altering neuroendocrine secretions and levels in the body, thereby changing this balance and increasing susceptibility to disease agents.

Animal experiments have shown that stressful social circumstances alter neural, hormonal, and immunologic control systems and lead to disease consequences (Ader et al., 1963; Calhoun, 1962; Gross, 1972; Ratcliffe, 1968). In human populations this series of links has not been established in any single study, though depressed lymphocyte function has been reported after bereavement (Bartrop et al., 1977). In cancer patients both cell-mediated and humoral immunity are frequently depressed. Furthermore, different hormonal patterns have been reported in patients with cancer of the breast and prostate (Henderson, Gerkins, and Pike (1975), and it is possible that some estrogens and androgens are responsive to stress (Lemon, 1969).

There is more animal, laboratory, and clinical evidence correlating social attachments (or the lack of them) with cardiovascular disease, particularly sudden death (Bovard, 1959; Buell and Eliot, 1979; Engel, 1971; Lown et al., 1980; Raab, 1966; Ratcliffe, 1968; Wolf, 1969). The pathways most often invoked as links are sympathetic-adrenomedullary responses, and a more slowly acting and hormonally mediated adreno-cortical response (Bovard, 1959, 1980). Physiological concomitants of increased sympathetic-adrenomedullary activity are (1) increased blood pressure and heart rate, (2) increased myocardial oxygen utilization, (3) increasing circulating levels of epinephrine and norepinephrine, (4) increased concentrations of plasma free fatty acids, and (5) increased plasma renin activity (Herd, 1979). In some cases, the role that social networks or social support may play is to inhibit a physiological response to stress. For example, individuals with an extended social network might have significantly lower resting pulse rates because of sympathetic inhibition than individuals without such support (Bovard, 1980). On the other hand, individuals faced with a sudden loss may experience increased sympathetic-adrenomedullary activity that could lead to the above-mentioned symptoms and consequently to sudden death.

Although the evidence linking social networks to specific disease-producing physiological responses is far from conclusive, it is clear that plausible pathways via a range of physiological responses do exist.

References

Ader R, Kreutner A, Jacobs HL: Social environment, emotionality and alloxan diabetes in the rat. *Psychosom. Med.* 25:60–68, 1963.

Antonovsky A: *Health, Stress and Coping*. San Francisco, Jossey-Bass, 1979.

Bahnson LB, Bahnson MB: Role of ego defenses: denial and repression in the etiology of malignant neoplasm. *Ann. N.Y. Acad. Sci.* 125:827–845, 1966.

Bartrop RW, Luckhurst E, Lazarus R, Kiloh LG, Penny R: Depressed lymphocyte function after bereavement. *Lancet* April 16, 1977, pp. 834–836.

Bell W, Boat MD: Urban neighborhoods and informal social relations. *Am. J. Sociol.* 62:391–398, 1957.

Bell W, Force M: Urban neighborhood types and participation in formal associations. *Am. Sociol. Rev.* 21:25–34, 1965.

Berkman LF: *Social Networks, Host Resistance, and Mortality: A Follow-up Study of Alameda County Residents*, doctoral thesis, University of California, Berkeley, 1977.

Berkman LF: Social network analysis and coronary heart disease. *Adv. Cardiol.* 29:37–49, 1982.

Block J: *The Challenge of Response Sets*. New York, Appleton-Century-Crofts, 1965.

Bott E: *Family and Social Networks*. New York, The Free Press, 1971.

Bovard E: The effects of social stimuli on the response to stress. *Psychol. Rev.* **66**:267–277, 1959.

Bovard E: Brain mechanisms in effects of social networks on viability. Unpublished manuscript, 1980.

Bradburn NM, Caplovitz D: *Reports on Happiness: A Pilot Study of Behavior Related to Mental Health.* Chicago, Aldine, 1965.

Brown GW, Bhrolchain MN, Harris T: Social class and psychiatric disturbance among women in an urban population. *Sociology.* **9**:225–254, 1975.

Buell J, Eliot RS: The role of emotional stress in the development of heart disease. *J.A.M.A.* **242**:365–368, 1979.

Calhoun JB: Population density and social pathology. *Sci. Amer.* **206**(2):139–148, 1962.

Cannon WB: Stresses and strains of homeostases. *Am. J. Med. Sci.* **189**:1–14, 1935.

Caplan R: *Organizational Stress and Individual Strain: A Social Psychological Study of Risk Factors in Coronary Heart Disease Among Administrators, Engineers and Scientists,* doctoral thesis, University of Michigan, Ann Arbor, 1971.

Carter H, Glick PC: *Marriage and Divorce: A Social and Economic Study.* American Public Health Association, Vital and Health Statistics, Cambridge, Mass., Harvard University Press, 1970.

Cassel J: The contribution of the social environment to host resistance. *Am. J. Epidemiol.* **104**(2):107–123, 1976.

Cobb S: Social support as a moderator of life stress. *Psychosom. Med.* **38**:300–314, 1976.

Comstock GW, Abbey H, Lundin FE: The nonofficial census as a basic tool for epidemiological observations in Washington County, Maryland, in Kessler II, Levin MC (eds): *The Community as an Epidemiologic Laboratory.* Baltimore, Johns Hopkins University Press, 1970, pp. 73–97.

Comstock GW, Partridge KP: Church attendance and health. *J. Chron. Dis.* **25**:665–672, 1972.

Cox PR, Ford JR: The mortality of widows shortly after widowhood. *Lancet* **1**:163–164, 1964.

Craven S, Wellman B: The network city. *Sociol. Enquiry* **43**:57–88, 1973.

Croog SH, Levine S: Religious identity and response to serious illness: a report on heart patients. *Soc. Sci. Med.* **6**:17–32, 1972.

Dean A, Lin N: The stress-buffering role of social support. *J. Nerv. Ment. Dis.* **165**:403–407, 1977.

DeAraujo G, Van Arsdel P, Holmes T, Dudley D: Life change, coping ability and chronic intrinsic asthma. *J. Psychosom. Res.* **17**:359–363, 1973.

Doehrman SR: Psycho-social aspects of recovery from coronary heart disease: a review. *Soc. Sci. Med.* **11**:199–218, 1977.

Dohrenwend BS, Dohrenwend BP: Some issues in research on stressful life events. *J. Nerv. Ment. Dis.* **166**:7–15, 1978.

Dubos R: *Man Adapting.* New Haven, Conn., Yale University Press.

Durkheim E: *Suicide.* New York, The Free Press, 1951.

Engel G: Sudden and rapid death during psychological stress. *Annls. Intern. Med.* **74**:771–782, 1971.

Finlayson A: Social networks as coping resources. *Soc. Sci. Med.* **10**:97–103, 1976.

Fischer A, Jackson R, Stueve C, Gerson K, Jones L: *Networks and Places: Social Relations in the Urban Setting.* New York, The Free Press, 1977.

Gans H: *The Urban Villagers.* Glencoe, Ill., The Free Press, 1962.

Goldberg E, Comstock G: Epidemiology of life events: frequency in general populations. *Am. J. Epidemiol.* 111:736–752, 1980.

Gordon R, Gordon K: Social factors in prevention of postpartum emotional problems, paper presented at American Orthospsychiatric Association Annual Meeting, Washington, D.C., 1967.

Gore S: The effect of social support in moderating the health consequences of unemployment. *J Health Soc. Behav.* 19:157–165, 1978.

Graham TW, Kaplan BH, Cornoni-Huntley JC, James SA, Becker C, Hames CF, Heyden S: Frequency of church attendance and blood pressure elevation. *J. Behav. Med.* 1:37–44, 1978.

Granovetter M: The strength of weak ties. *Am. J. Sociol.* 78:1360–1380, 1973.

Gross WB: Effect of social stress on occurrence of Marek's disease in chickens. *Am. J. Vet. Res.* 33(11):2275–2279, 1972.

Haynes RB, Sackett DL: A workshop symposium: compliance with therapeutic regimes—annotated bibliography. Dept. of Clinical Epidemiology and Biostatistics, McMaster University Medical Centre, Hamilton, Ont. 1974.

Helsing K, Szklo M: Mortality after bereavement. *Am J. Epidemiol.* 114:41–52, 1981.

Helsing K, Szklo M, Comstock G: Factors associated with mortality after widowhood. *Am. J. Public Health* 71:802–809, 1981.

Henderson BE, Gerkins VR, Pike MC: Sexual factors in pregnancy, in Fraumeni JF (ed): *Persons at High Risk of Cancer.* New York, Academic Press, 1975, pp. 267–284.

Henderson S, Byrne DG, Duncan-Jones P, Adcock S, Scott R, Steele GP: Social bonds in the epidemiology of neurosis: a preliminary communication. *Br. J. Psychiatry* 132:463–466, 1978.

Henderson S, Duncan-Jones P, Byrne DG, Scott R, Adcock S: Social bonds, adversity and neurosis. Presented at the World Psychiatric Assoc. Section Committee on Epidemiology and Community Psychiatry Triennal meeting, St. Louis, October 1978a.

Herd A: Behavioral factors in the physiological mechanisms of cardiovascular disease. Paper presented at First Annual Meeting on Behavioral Medicine Research, Snowbird, Utah, 1979.

Hochstim JR, Renne KS: Reliability of response in a sociomedical population study. *Public Opinion Q.* 35:69–79, 1971.

Holmes TH, Rahe RH: The social readjustment rating scale. *J. Psychosom. Res.* 11:213–218, 1967.

House JS, Wells JA: Occupational stress, social support and health, in McLean A, Black G, Colligan M (eds): *Reducing Occupational Stress: Proceedings of a Conference.* USDHEW (NIOSH) Publ. No. 78–140, 1978, pp. 8–29.

Hyman MD: Social isolation and performance in rehabilitation. *J. Chron. Dis.* 25:85–97, 1972.

Jenkins CD, Rosenman RH, Zyzanski SJ: Prediction of clinical coronary disease by a test for coronary-prone behavior pattern. *N. Engl. J. Med.* 290:1271–1316, 1974.

Joseph J: *Social Affiliation, Risk Factor Status, and Coronary Heart Disease: A Cross-Sectional Study of Japanese-American Men,* doctoral thesis, University of California, Berkeley, 1980.

Kaplan BH, Cassel JC, Gore S: Social support and health. *Med. Care* (Suppl.) 15(5):47–58, 1977.

Koskenvuo M, Kaprio J, Kesaniemi A, Sarna S: Differences in mortality from ischemic heart disease by marital status and social class. *J. Chron. Dis.* 33:95–106, 1980.

Kraus S, Lilienfeld AM: Some epidemiologic aspects of the high mortality rates in the young widowed group. *J. Chron. Dis.* 10:207–217, 1959.

Laumann E: *Bonds of Pluralism: The Form and Substance of Urban Social Networks.* New York, John Wiley & Sons, 1973.

Lazarus RS, Cohen JB: Environmental stress, in Altman I, Wohlwill JF (eds): *Human Behaviors and Environment. Advances in Theory and Research,* Vol. 2. New York, Plenum Press, 1976, pp. 89–127.

Lazarus RS, Speisman JL, Mordkoff AM, Davidson LA: A laboratory study of psychological stress produced by a motion picture film. *Psychol. Monogr.* 76(34): Whole No. 553, 1962.

Lee NH: *The Search for an Abortionist.* Chicago, University of Chicago Press, 1969.

Lemon HM: Endocrine influences on human mammary cancer formation. *Cancer* 23:781–790, 1969.

LeShan L: An emotional life-history pattern associated with neoplastic disease. *Ann. N.Y. Acad. Sci.* 125:780–793, 1966.

Liebow E: *Talley's Corner.* Boston, Little, Brown, 1967.

Litman TJ: The family and physical rehabilitation. *J. Chron. Dis.* 19:211–217, 1966.

Litwak E: Occupational mobility and extended family cohesion. *Am. Sociol. Rev.* 25:9–21, 1960.

Lowenthal MJ, Haven C: Interaction and adaptation: intimacy as a critical variable. *Am. Sociol. Rev.* 33:20–30, 1967.

Lown B, Desilva R, Reich P, Murawski B: Psychophysiologic factors in sudden cardiac death. *Am. J. Psychiatry* 127:1325–1335, 1980.

Maddison D, Viola A: The health of widows in the year following bereavement. *J. Psychosom. Res.* 12:297–306, 1968.

Marmot MG, Syme SL: Acculturation and coronary heart disease in Japanese-Americans. *Am. J. Epidemiol.* 104:225–247, 1976.

Marris P: *Widows and Their Families.* London, Routledge & Kegan Paul, 1958.

McCloskey H, Schaar JH: Psychological dimensions of anomy. *Am. Sociol. Rev.* 30:14–40, 1965.

McKinlay J: Social network influence in morbid episodes and the career of help seeking, in Eisenberg L, Kleinman A (eds): *The Relevance of Social Science for Medicine.* Dordrecht, Reidel, 1980, pp. 77–107.

McKinlay JB: Social networks, lay consultation and help-seeking behaviors. *Social Forces* 51:275–292, 1973.

McNeil D: *Mortality Among the Widows in Connecticut.* MPH Essay, Yale University, New Haven, Conn., 1973.

Medalie JH, Kahn HA, Neufeld HN, Riss E, Goldbourt U: Five-year myocardial infarction incidence—II. Association of single variables to age and birth-place. *J. Chron. Dis.* 26:329–349, 1973.

Mitchell JC: The concept and use of social networks, in Mitchell JC (ed): *Social Networks in Urban Situations.* Manchester, England, Manchester University Press, 1969, pp. 1–50.

Mueller D: Social networks: a promising direction for research of the relationship of the social environment to psychiatric disorder. *Soc. Sci. Med.* 14:147–161, 1980.

Mueller D, Edwards DW, Yarvis RM: Stressful life events and psychiatric symptomatology: change or undesirability. *J. Health Soc. Behav.* 18:307–316, 1977.

Naguib SM, Geiser PB, Comstock GW: Responses to a program of screening for cervical cancer. *Public Health Rep.* 83:990–998, 1968.

Nichaman MZ, Hamilton HB, Kegan A, Sacks ST, Syme SL: Epidemiologic studies of coronary disease and stroke: distribution of biochemical risk factors. *Am. J. Epidemiol.* 102:491–501, 1975.

Nuckolls KB, Cassel JC, Kaplan BH: Psychosocial assets, life crisis, and prognosis of pregnancy. *Am. J. Epidemiol.* 95:431–441, 1972.

Ortmeyer CF: Variations in mortality, morbidity, and health care by marital status, in Erhardt LL, Berlin JE (eds): *Mortality and Morbidity in the United States.* Cambridge, Mass., Harvard University Press, 1974, pp. 159–188.

Parkes CM: The effects of bereavement on physical and mental health—a study of medical records of widows. *Br. Med. J.* 2:274–279, 1964.

Parkes CM, Benjamin B, Fitzgerald BG: A broken heart: a statistical study of increased mortality among widows. *Br. Med. J.* 1:740–743, 1969.

Phillips DL: Mental health status, social participation, and happiness. *J. Health Soc. Behav.* 8:285–291, 1967.

Raab W: Emotional and sensory stress factors in myocardial pathology. *Am. Heart J.* 72:538–564, 1966.

Rabkin JG, Struening EL: Life events, stress, and illness. *Science* 194:1013–1020, 1976.

Ratcliffe HL: Environment, behavior and disease, in Stellar E , Sprague JM (eds.): *Progress in Physiological Psychology.* New York, Academic Press, 1968, pp. 161–228.

Rees WP, Lutkins SG: Mortality of bereavement. *Br. Med. J.* 4:13–16, 1967.

Rosenman RH, Brand RJ, Sholtz RI, Friedman M: Multivariate protection of coronary heart disease during 8-½ year follow-up in western collaborative study. *Am. J. Cardiol.* 37:903–910, 1976.

Rotter J: Generalized expectancies for internal versus external control of reinforcement. *Psychological Monograph* 80(1), Whole No. 609, 1966.

Satariano W, Syme SL: Life change and disease: coping with change, in McGaugh, JL, Kiesler S (eds): *Aging: Biology and Behavior.* New York, Academic Press, 1981, pp. 311–328.

Schacter S: *Psychology of Affiliation.* Palo Alto, Calif., Stanford University Press, 1959.

Schmale A, Iker IT: The psychological setting of uterine cervical cancer. *Ann. N.Y. Acad. Sci.* 125:794–801, 1966.

Segal B, Phillips D, Feldmesser R: Social integration, emotions, adjustment and illness behavior. *Social Forces* 46:237–246, 1967.

Seligman M: *Helplessness.* San Francisco, W.H. Freeman, 1975.

Selye H: *The Stress of Life.* New York, McGraw-Hill, 1956.

Shuval JT, Antonovsky A, Davies AM: *Social Functions of Medical Practice.* San Francisco, Jossey-Bass, 1970.

Sosa R, Kennel J, Klaus M: The effect of a supportive companion on perinatal problems, length of labor and mother-infant interaction. *N. Engl. J. Med.* 303:597–600, 1980.

Stack CB: *All Our Kin: Strategies for Survival in a Black Community.* New York, Harper & Row, 1974.

Suchman EA: Health orientation and medical care. *Am. J. Public Health* **56**:97–105, 1966.

Susser M: Widowhood: a statistical life stress or a stressful life event. *Am. J. Public Health* **71**:793–795, 1981.

Syme SL, Berkman LF: Social class, susceptibility, and sickness. *Am. J. Epidemiol.* **104**:1–8, 1976.

Theorell T, Lind E, Floderus G: The relationship of disturbing life changes and emotions to the early development of myocardial infarction and other serious illnesses. *Int. J. Epidemiol.* **4**:281–293, 1975.

Thiel HG, Parker D, Bruce T: Stress factors and the risk of myocardial infarction. *Psychol. Res.* **17**:43–57, 1973.

Thoits PA: Conceptual, methodological, and theoretical problems in studying social support as a buffer against life stress. *J. Health Soc. Behav.* **23**:145–158, 1982.

Tilly C: An interactional scheme for analysis of communities, cities, and urbanization, manuscript, Dept. of Sociology, University of Michigan, Ann Arbor, 1972.

Valentine CA: *Culture and Poverty.* Chicago, University of Chicago Press, 1968.

Walker NK, MacBride A, Vachon ML: Social support networks and the crisis of bereavement. *Soc. Sci. Med.* **11**:35–41, 1977.

Wechsler H, Pugh TF: Fit of individual and community characteristics and rates of psychiatric hospitalization. *Am. J. Sociol.* **73**:331–338, 1967.

Weiss NS: Marital status and risk factors for coronary heart disease: the United States Health Examination Survey of Adults. *Br. J. Prev. Soc. Med.* **27**:41–43, 1973.

Wellman B: Applying network analyses to the study of support, in Gottlieb BH (ed): *Social Networks and Social Support.* Beverly Hills, Calif., Sage Publications, 1981, pp. 171–200.

Whitten N, Wolfe A: Network analysis, in Honigman JJ (ed): *The Handbook of Social and Cultural Anthropology.* Chicago, Rand-McNally, 1974, pp. 717–746.

Whyte WF: *Street Corner Society: The Social Structure of an Italian Slum.* Chicago, University of Chicago Press, 1955.

Winkelstein W, Kegan A, Kato H, Sacks ST: Epidemiologic studies of coronary heart disease and stroke in Japanese men living in Japan, Hawaii, and California: blood pressure distributions. *Am. J. Epidemiol.* **102**:502–513, 1975.

Wolf S: Psychosocial forces in myocardial infarction and sudden death. *Circulation* **4**(Suppl.):74–83, 1969.

Wolff HG: *Stress and Disease.* Springfield, Ill.: Charles C Thomas, 1953.

5. A multivariate analysis of health practices and social networks

DEBORAH WINGARD   LISA F. BERKMAN

Introduction

Chapters 3 and 4 present evidence of the substantial correlation between mortality and both health practices and social networks, which persists after controlling individually for a wide range of factors. However, the methods used for the analyses described in those chapters permitted examining only a few variables in any single analysis. For instance, health practices were found to be associated with mortality while holding constant age, sex, and a third variable of interest, such as health status. Many variables identified as potential confounders were, however, associated with both predictor and outcome variables. Although in all cases independent relationships were found between health practices, social networks, and mortality risk, it does seem possible that, cumulatively, the confounders might account for a great deal of the relationship between health practices, social networks, and mortality risk.

In order to consider that issue, it was necessary to examine the role that predictor variables play in determining mortality risk while simultaneously controlling for many potentially confounding factors. In addition, we wished to assess more accurately the independent contribution to mortality risk made by each of the health practices and the components of the Social Network Index. We were also interested in the relationship between social networks and health practices, and the cumulative impact these two sets of factors would have on mortality risk.

A method well suited to these needs is multiple logistic analysis. By using a multiple logistic model and the usual age-adjusted analyses, it is possible to examine many questions that were not considered in Chapters 3 and 4. Therefore, this chapter focuses on exactly the same variables in the same population used in previous chapters, but they are explored with a different method.

Methods

Statistical analyses

Three types of examinations are included in this chapter: (1) multiple logistic analyses in which approximate relative mortality risks among Alameda County residents aged 30–69 years in 1965 are obtained while controlling for several variables simultaneously (Rosenman et al., 1976); (2) a decile of risk analysis developed by Hudes (1980); and (3) as presented in Chapters 3 and 4, sex-specific 9-year mortality rates, age adjusted by the indirect method with Mantel-Haenszel (1959) chi-square tests of significance as modified by Brand and Sholtz (1976) to adjust for more than two categories of a given variable. The multiple logistic approach will be described in some detail because it is the principal method used in this chapter.

In the multiple logistic risk model, the mortality risk (R) for k risk factors $(x_1, x_2 \ldots x_k)$ is represented by the equation:

$$R = \frac{1}{1 + \exp - (B_0 + B_1 x_1 + \ldots + B_k x_k)}$$

The logistic coefficients $(B_0, B_1 \ldots B_k)$ are estimated by the method of maximum likelihood. Discriminant analysis (Truett et al., 1967) is used to provide initial values, followed by Gauss-Newton iteration (Walker and Duncan, 1967). The quantity $\ln (R/1 - R)$ is called the logit of R and is the transformation from which this model derives its name.

An approximate relative risk (odds ratio) per unit change in level of risk factor x_i, is e^{B_i}. More generally, $e^{(Dx_i B_i)}$ approximates the relative risk per D units of change in the level of risk factor, x_i, and can be used to determine the relative risk of the highest versus the lowest category of a variable.

The multiple logistic risk model assumes that any multicategorical factor as scaled in the analysis is associated with the dependent variable in a logistic manner. Therefore, a preliminary, univariate analysis of the mortality risk of each multicategorical variable is conducted. If the pattern of the mortality risk associated with each successive category of the variable does not follow a logistic curve, that variable is not included in its multicategorical form. In such a case, when a likelihood ratio test of the logistic pattern is rejected at $P \leq 0.20$, the scaled variable is replaced by a collection of dichotomous variables—one for each subcategory except for one set aside as a reference subcategory. In the present analysis, two multicategorical variables, use of preventive health services and physical health status, are replaced by appropriate dichotomous variables.

Although the multiple logistic model determines the independent relative risk of each health practice or social network component, it should be noted that this analysis allows only a general comparison of these variables. Each relative risk is dependent on the categorization of that variable. A different cutpoint for alcohol consumption, for example, might yield a different relative risk. In addition, care must be taken when comparing relative risks of differently categorized variables. Given the above restrictions, approximate relative risks for dichotomous variables can be directly compared, whereas standardized odds ratios are probably most appropriate when comparing continuous variables. Comparing relative risks of dichotomous and multicategorical variables can provide only a qualitative comparison. (See Rosenman et al., 1976, for a fuller discussion of this problem.)

The multiple logistic risk model also imposes definite constraints on risk patterns that can emerge from data analysis. To assess the goodness of fit of the model to the data, observed and expected numbers of deaths are compared after grouping subjects by decile of estimated risk. This provides some indication of the adequacy of the model for multivariate prediction.

Variables studied

In this chapter, seven health practices (physical activity, smoking status, weight status, alcohol consumption, sleeping patterns, eating breakfast, and snacking between meals) and the four components of the Social Network Index (marital status, contacts with friends and relatives, and church and group membership) are analyzed by the multiple logistic model. They are categorized as they were in the two summary scales, the Health Practices and Social Network Indices. The first five of the health practices and three of the four network components are dichotomized. The two health practices concerning eating habits and one set of questions about contacts with friends and relatives are divided into three categories. The summary Health Practices and Social Network Indices are used in the forms described in Chapters 3 and 4. In addition, seven demographic and social variables implicated as mortality risk factors and associated with health practices and social networks are controlled for in these analyses. Included are age, sex, race, socioeconomic status, physical health status, use of preventive health services, and life satisfaction. Classification of each is presented in Table 5-1.

Table 5-1. Classification of variables influencing mortality, 1965–1974

Variable	Categories	Remarks
Health practices		
Physical activity (0, 1)	Active, inactive	Based on the frequency (often, sometimes, never) and presumed strenuousness of leisure-time participation in active sports, swimming or long walks, physical exercise, gardening, and/or hunting or fishing
Smoking status (0, 1)	Never, ever	Cigarettes
Weight status (0, 1)	Average (9.9% underweight to 29.9% overweight), underweight or overweight	Measured by Quetelet Index (weight in pounds height in inches)^2, categories based on Metropolitan Life Insurance reports of desirable weights (1959)
Alcohol consumption (0, 1)	Low, high drinking index	Based on frequency of drinking (number of times per week) and amount consumed (usual number of drinks at a sitting) for beer, wine, and liquor combined, dichotomization based on studies of drinking practices by Cahalan and Cisin (1968)
Sleeping patterns (0, 1)	7 or 8 hrs/night, ≤ 6 or ≥ 9 hrs/night	Based on usual number of hours slept per night
Eating breakfast (1–3)	Often, sometimes, never	
Snacking (1–3)	Never, sometimes, often	
Health Practices Index (1–3)	0–2, 3, 4–5 high-risk practices	See Chapter 3 for details.
Social networks[a]		
Marital status (1, 2)	Currently married, all other	
Contacts with friends and relatives (1–3)	Many, some, few	Based on three questions about how many friends and relatives a person has, and how often they are seen
Church membership (1, 2)	Member, nonmember	
Group membership (1, 2)	Member, nonmember	
Social Network Index (1–4)	Four groups, no or few contacts to many contacts	Based on above four components; see Chapter 4 for details
Potential confounders[b]		
Age (30–69)	Years	
Sex (1, 2)	Female, male	
Race (0, 1)	White, black, other	
Socioeconomic status (1–5)	Five groups, high to low class	Based on education and household income

Table 5-1. (Continued)

Variable	Categories	Remarks
Physical health status (1–4)	No health problem, symptom, chronic condition, disability	Derived from extensive checklist of health problems, coded by most serious condition reported (Belloc et al., 1971)
Use of preventive health services (1–3)	Visits doctor and dentist, visits doctor *or* dentists, no visits to either	Based on visits to a doctor or dentist when not ill
Life satisfaction (1–3)	Highly satisfied, satisfied, dissatisfied	Based on nine questions about satisfaction with aspects of one's life, such as marriage or job

[a]Based on Berkman and Syme (1979).
[b]Based on Berkman (1977).

The multiple logistic model and 9-year mortality risk of individual health practices and social networks

Our first task was to assess the independent impact of each health practice and type of social tie on mortality risk. This was done in order to ascertain whether the results presented in Chapters 3 and 4 would be confirmed by more elaborate analyses. In two separate logistic analyses, seven health practices and four different kinds of social ties were examined while controlling for age and sex to see if they would predict mortality risk independently of each other.

Health practices

Approximate relative mortality risks were calculated for each of the seven health practices and for two potentially confounding variables, age and sex, by multiple logistic analysis. These are presented in Table 5-2 along with the logistic coefficients and significance probabilities. Five of the health practices reveal substantial and statistically significant mortality risks, cigarette smoking and physical activity having the highest relative risks in these analyses. However, it is important to remember that different categorizations of the variables might influence their relative ranking. The results are similar to those obtained from the univariate analyses in Chapter 3, where in each case the association of physical activity, smoking status, weight status, alcohol consumption, and sleeping pattern with mortality were statistically significant for at least one sex.

Table 5-2. Nine-year mortality risk of individual health practices, multiple logistic analysis, 1965–1974

	Approximate relative mortality risk		
Variable (high/low risk category)	Logistic coefficient	Relative risk[a]	Significance probability
Health practices			
Physical activity (inactive/active)	0.5488	1.7	< 0.001
Smoking status (ever/never)	0.7018	2.0	< 0.001
Weight status (abnormal/normal)	0.3105	1.4	0.02
Alcohol consumption (high/low)	0.4057	1.5	0.01
Sleeping pattern (≤ 6 or $\geq 9/7$ or 8 hrs)	0.4746	1.6	< 0.001
Eating breakfast (never/often)	0.0054	1.1	0.95
Snacking (often/never)	0.0742	1.2	0.34
Potential confounders			
Age (69/30 years)	0.0912	35.0	< 0.001
Sex (male/female)	0.4237	1.5	< 0.001
Intercept	8.6728		

[a]Approximate relative mortality risk (odds ratio for high- compared to low-risk category.

The results indicate that the five practices have an impact on mortality independently of each other. For example, the analysis signifies that whereas physical activity may have an effect on mortality through weight control or smoking cessation, it has a sizeable direct effect on mortality risk that is independent of those other factors. This is also true of each of the other four above-mentioned health practices.

The relative mortality risks associated with eating breakfast and snacking between meals are smaller than the others and statistically nonsignificant in the multiple logistic analysis of the experience of men and women between the ages 30 and 69 ($P = 0.95$ and 0.34, respectively). As in the analyses presented in Chapter 3, these two variables do not appear to exert a substantial or independent effect on mortality risk. Again, it should be noted that these results do not indicate that eating practices are unimportant; the items in the questionnaire, the limitation to persons 30–69 years of age, the categorization of the variables, and the form of analysis may have contributed to failure to find a statistically significant relationship.

In addition, approximate relative mortality risks for various combinations of health practices can be determined from the information in Table 5-2. For example, to determine the relative risk associated with physical inactivity and smoking, calculate the natural antilogarithm of the sum of their logistic coefficients: $e^{(0.5488 + 0.7018)} = 3.5$. Thus a person who is both inactive and smokes cigarettes has 3.5 times the 9-year mortality risk of a physically active nonsmoker.

Social networks

Table 5-3 shows the approximate relative mortality risks for the four components of the Social Network Index and two potentially confounding variables (age and sex), as determined by a multiple logistic analysis. Of the four types of social contact, three (marital status, contacts with friends and relatives, and church membership) have statistically significant, independent relationships to mortality risk. Group membership had a weaker association with mortality risk—an association that fails to reach conventional statistical significance $(P = 0.25)$. These findings differ slightly from the univariate analyses in which all four components of the Social Network Index were significantly associated with mortality for at least one sex $(P \leq 0.05)$. In those analyses group membership showed a stronger and significant relationship to mortality among women in the sample.

The independent relationships of most of the network components to mortality add to the findings presented in Chapter 4. Those results indicated that increasing social isolation—that is, missing several kinds of social contact—was more important than any single missing tie in predicting increased mortality risk. These multiple logistic findings suggest that beyond mounting general isolation, the lack of *specific* kinds of ties may have a negative relationship to health.

Table 5-3. Nine-year mortality risk of components of the Social Network Index, multiple logistic analysis, 1965–1974

Variable (high/low risk category)	Approximate relative mortality risk		
	Logistic coefficient	Relative risk[a]	Significance probability
Social networks			
Marital status (unmarried/married)	0.3947	1.5	< 0.001
Contacts with friends and relatives (few/many)	0.3499	2.0	< 0.001
Church membership (nonmember/member)	0.3014	1.4	0.02
Group membership (nonmember/member)	0.1399	1.2	0.25
Potential confounders			
Age (69/30 years)	0.0875	30.3	< 0.001
Sex (male/female)	0.5550	1.7	< 0.001
Intercept	−9.6289		

[a]Approximate relative mortality risk (odds ratio) for high- compared to low-risk category.

Joint contribution of health practices
and social networks to mortality risk

Nine-year mortality risk of health practices
and social networks: age-adjusted rates

Variations in health practices among persons with differing social networks conceivably could explain the observed association between the
Social Network Index and mortality. For example, unmarried persons
with few living relatives or friends may smoke cigarettes more frequently
or drink more alcohol than married persons with many friends and
relatives. Alternatively, persons who rarely join in any group activity may
rarely partake in physical activity. Such associations may be coincidental,
or may be a result of personality or ill health.

To determine if health practices and social networks predict mortality
independently from one another, age-adjusted mortality rates are examined for the Health Practice Index within each category of the Social
Network Index, and vice versa. The results are presented in Table 5-4.

A clear gradient in mortality rates is seen for the Health Practices Index
in every category of the Social Network Index, except for men reporting
the least connections. The chi-square value for the differences in mortality
rates by health practices when adjusting for both age and social networks
is highly significant ($P \leq 0.001$) for both men and women. This analysis
indicates that health practices are associated with mortality, independent
from the effects of social networks.

A mortality gradient is also seen for the Social Network Index within
most categories of the Health Practices Index. Again, the principal exception is among men, this time for those scoring the lowest on the Health
Practices Index. The chi-square value for the differences in mortality rates
by social networks when adjusting for both age and health practices is
also significant ($P \leq 0.01$) for both men and women. Therefore, social
networks appear to be associated with mortality, independent from the
effects of health practices.

Interaction between health practices and social networks is not readily
apparent for men, but may exist for women in this population. Note that
among women the relative mortality risk associated with the Health
Practices Index is higher among persons reporting the weakest social
network ($20.2/4.9 = 4.1$) than among those reporting the strongest
($7.2/3.0 = 2.4$). Likewise, the relative mortality risk associated with the
Social Network Index is highest among women scoring low on the Health
Practice Index ($20.2/7.2 = 2.8$) and lowest among those scoring high
($4.9/3.0 = 1.6$). In addition, the relative risk associated with scoring low
on both indices ($20.2/3.0 = 6.7$) is greater than the sum of the age-adjusted

Table 5-4. Age-adjusted mortality rates from all causes (per 100) by health practices and social networks, 1965–1974

Health Practices Index	Social Network Index								
	I[a]	(N)	II	(N)	III	(N)	IV	(N)	Total	(N)
Men									
Low	15.4	(56)	18.7	(143)	13.4	(114)	15.4	(91)	16.0	(404)
Medium	23.2	(51)	14.9	(203)	9.2	(246)	6.9	(248)	10.9	(748)
High	7.9	(51)	6.4	(259)	6.4	(342)	4.8	(425)	5.8	(1077)
Total	15.6	(158)	12.3	(605)	8.6	(702)	6.9	(764)	9.5	(2229)
Women									
Low	20.2	(78)	11.8	(181)	7.8	(95)	7.2	(72)	11.9	(426)
Medium	11.2	(113)	7.8	(271)	4.7	(203)	5.8	(222)	7.1	(809)
High	4.9	(85)	4.7	(408)	3.8	(304)	3.0	(464)	3.9	(1261)
Total	12.1	(276)	7.3	(860)	4.9	(602)	4.3	(758)	6.4	(2496)

[a]Social Network Index ranges from I (least connections) to IV (most connections).

relative risks for each index alone $(11.9/3.9 + 12.1/4.3 = 5.8)$. Therefore, the interaction of social networks and health practices among women may be synergistic as opposed to additive. These associations do not hold for men, possibly because of the earlier noted exceptions in mortality gradients among persons scoring low on either index, or because of interactions with other variables such as physical health status.

This analysis indicates that the Social Network and Health Practices Indices are associated with mortality independent from one another, and that people who have both weak networks and high risk health practices are much more likely to die during the follow-up period than those with strong networks and low risk health practices.

Nine-year mortality risk of health practices and social networks: multiple logistic model

The mortality risk associated with the Health Practices and Social Network Indices shown in Table 5-4 may reflect associations with other variables, such as race, socioeconomic status, or physical health status. Chapters 3 and 4 demonstrate that each index is associated with mortality independently of these variables, although they also influence the degree of mortality risk. To determine if the Health Practices and Social Network Indices predict mortality independently of the joint effect of these other known mortality risk factors, as well as each other, two multiple logistic analyses are presented in Table 5-5, one for men and one for women.

Table 5-5. Nine-year mortality risk of health practices and social networks, detailed results for two multiple logistic analyses, 1965–1974

| Variable (codes) | Approximate relative mortality risk[a] | | | | | |
| | Men | | | Women | | |
	Coef.	RR	P	Coef.	RR	P
Health Practices Index (1–3)	0.4429	2.4	<0.001	0.3952	2.2	<0.001
Social Network Index (1–4)	0.2574	2.2	0.002	0.2856	2.4	0.001
Potential confounders						
Age (30–69)	0.0915	35.5	<0.001	0.0679	14.1	<0.001
Race (0, 1)	0.0606	1.1	0.79	0.4262	1.5	0.06
Socioeconomic status (1–5)	0.0461	1.2	0.55	0.0837	1.4	0.34
Physical health status (compared to healthy)						
Symptoms (0, 1)	0.1751	1.2	0.48	−0.3788	0.7	0.23
Chronic conditions (0, 1)	0.2100	1.2	0.33	0.0841	1.1	0.75
Disability (0, 1)	1.4374	4.2	<0.001	0.7779	2.2	0.01
Use of preventive health services (compared to often)						
Sometimes (0, 1)	0.1780	1.2	0.35	−0.0374	1.0	0.86
Rarely (0, 1)	0.2512	1.3	0.24	0.0662	1.1	0.77
Life satisfaction (1–3)	−0.0008	1.0	0.99	0.3246	1.4	0.01
Intercept	−9.0590	—	—	−8.7375	—	—

[a]Abbreviations : Coef., Logistic coefficient; RR, approximate relative mortality risk (odds ratio) for highest compared to lowest risk category; P, significance probability.

The Health Practices Index and the Social Network Index are each associated with a more than twofold excess mortality risk, which is statistically significant for men and women $(P \leq 0.001)$. Both indices predict mortality independently of each other, and also independently of age, race, socioeconomic status, physical health, use of preventive health services, and self-assessment of life satisfaction.

Table 5-5 also illustrates a relationship between disability and mortality risk for both men and women, and an independent association between life satisfaction and mortality for women but not for men.

Nine-year mortality risk and individual adjustment for eight other variables

To determine how each potentially confounding variable influences the mortality risk associated with health practices and social networks, two series of 11 multivariate analyses are presented in Tables 5-6 (for health practices) and 5-7 (for social networks). The first line in each table shows

Table 5-6. Changes in the relative mortality risk for the Health Practices Index with adjustment (11 multiple logistic analyses), 1965–1974

Adjustment variables	Approximate relative mortality risk[a]
Unadjusted	3.52
Sex	3.50
Age	3.42
Age, sex	3.41
Age, sex, race	3.32
Age, sex, socioeconomic status	3.35
Age, sex, use of preventive health services	3.31
Age, sex, life satisfaction	3.08
Age, sex, physical health status	2.73
Age, sex, Social Network Index	3.00
All eight variables	2.31

[a]For the highest compared to the lowest risk category of the Health Practices Index.

the approximate relative mortality risk for either health practices or social network without adjusting for *any* covariables. In the second line, sex is considered as a covariable; in the third, age is considered, and so on until all eight potentially confounding variables are individually considered. This series of analyses indicates to what extent each of the eight variables accounts for the relationship between mortality and health practices on the one hand, and social networks on the other.

HEALTH PRACTICES

As seen in Table 5-6, persons with four or five high-risk health practices were 3.5 times more likely to die during the follow-up period than persons with zero to two high-risk health practices when no adjustment is made for other variables. When each covariable is added to the analysis, the relative mortality risk associated with the Health Practices Index is reduced, indicating that persons scoring low on this index tend to have other high-risk characteristics.

Adjustment for physical health status in 1965 reduces the relative mortality risk associated with the Health Practices Index more than any other variable in this analysis. Apparently persons in poor physical health were more likely to have high-risk health practices than persons in good health. Whether poor health causes high-risk behavior, such as physical inactivity, or such behavior causes poor health, is not deducible from this analysis. Data presented in Chapter 6, however, suggest that risk behavior does

Table 5-7. Changes in the relative mortality risk for the Social Network Index with adjustment (11 multiple logistic analyses), 1965–1974

Adjustment variables	Approximate relative mortality risk[a]
Unadjusted	2.83
Sex	3.10
Age	2.62
Age, sex	2.96
Age, sex, race	2.97
Age, sex, socioeconomic status	2.88
Age, sex, use of preventive health services	2.86
Age, sex, life satisfaction	2.54
Age, sex, physical health status	2.63
Age, sex, Health Practices Index	2.36
All eight variables	2.14

[a]For the highest compared to the lowest risk category of the Social Network Index.

influence changes in physical health status. Adjustment for all eight factors, including 1965 physical health status, reduces the overall risk from 3.5 to 2.3.

SOCIAL NETWORKS

Similarly, to determine how each potentially confounding variable influences the mortality risk associated with social networks, a series of 11 multivariate analyses are presented in Table 5-7. The relative risk of mortality associated with the Social Network Index is reduced or unchanged by adjustment for every factor except sex. The increase that comes with adjustment for sex reflects the fact that women, who normally are at a lower risk of death than men, are more likely than men to score low on the Social Network Index. The latter is verified by data presented in Chapter 4.

Adjustment for the Health Practices Index reduces the relative mortality risk associated with the Social Network Index more than any other variable in this analysis. Apparently, persons with high-risk health practices were more likely to have few social connections. Again, it is not possible to determine if one causes the other or if both reflect some other high-risk characteristic. In this analysis it is noteworthy that physical health status has less impact on the reduction of mortality risk in the social network than in the health practices analysis. In all, adjustment for the eight variables reduces the overall mortality risk from 2.8 to 2.1.

Appropriateness of the multiple logistic model

To assess the goodness of fit of the multiple logistic model to the data, observed and expected numbers of deaths are compared after grouping subjects by decile of estimated risk. This provides some indication of the adequacy of the model for multivariate prediction. Figure 5-1 demonstrates a generally good agreement between observed and expected death in each decile of risk.

Discussion

The multivariate analyses in this chapter indicate that the Social Network and Health Practices Indices are each associated with mortality risk independently of one another and of seven other potential confounders. In addition, most individual health practices and components of the Social Network Index are independently associated with mortality risk. This verifies the relationships originally demonstrated by univariate analyses in Chapters 3 and 4. In addition, the logistic analyses reveal that of all

Fig. 5-1. Goodness of fit of the multiple logistic model to the data: Deciles of risk, Alameda County, 1965–1974.

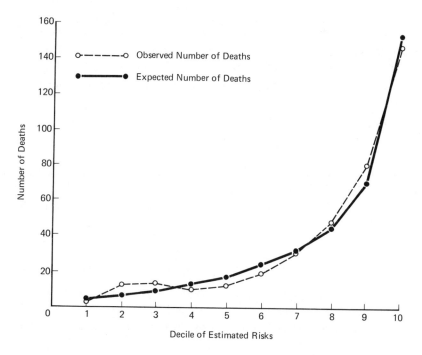

the potential confounders considered, physical health status has the greatest influence on the mortality risk associated with the Health Practices Index. On the other hand, the mortality risk associated with the Social Network Index is affected most by the Health Practice Index.

The age-adjusted analysis (in Table 5-4) further suggests that health practices and social networks may interact synergistically. For women, the relative risk associated with scoring low on both indices is greater than the sum of their age-adjusted relative risks (6.7 versus 5.8). Synergism is also seen in the multiple logistic analysis, for the model assumes a multiplicate interaction (i.e., relative risk) between variables. Although it is possible to use interaction terms to determine if any interaction greater than this is present, such synergism was not assessed in this chapter.

An association disclosed in a univariate analysis may be a direct association, or it may be indirect through another variable. In the latter case, multivariate analysis that includes this other variable will reduce or eliminate the association. Whatever association remains after adjustment may be a direct (independent) association. However, even when an association is reduced or eliminated, that variable could still be important etiologically to health. What matters is whether the indirect association reflects a coincidental or causal relationship involving the other variable. For example, the univariate association of alcohol consumption and mortality in Chapter 3 may be coincidental, reflecting smoking habits. Research has demonstrated that persons who consume moderate to large amounts of alcohol also tend to be smokers (Cahalan et al., 1969). Thus the high mortality rates among alcohol consumers could conceivably be entirely a result of smoking habits. The multivariate analysis in Table 5-2 suggests, however, that the association between alcohol consumption and mortality includes some pathways that do not involve smoking, because adjustment for smoking, as well as for other health practices, for age, and for sex, reduces but does not eliminate the risk of mortality.

Indirect relationships are not all coincidental, but may reflect causal associations with a third variable. For example, the mortality risk associated with physical inactivity in Chapter 3 is reduced after adjustment in Table 5-2 for other health practices, such as weight status. Although these variables could represent a coincidental relationship, they may also reflect indirect causal relationships. Physical activity may induce weight loss, which in turn lowers mortality risk. In this case, physical activity would be indirectly associated with mortality risk by causing changes in another risk factor. Weight loss would be the more proximate cause.

Two health practices, eating breakfast and snacking between meals, showed a small association with mortality after multivariate adjustment. This suggests that the weak association with mortality seen in Chapter 3 may possibly be indirect, involving the other variables. It is also possible that the variables used do not measure significant aspects of eating.

One component of the Social Network Index, group membership, likewise shows no significant association with mortality after multivariate adjustment. In earlier analyses this variable was significantly related to mortality risk among women but not among men. The weak association found in the logistic analyses may reflect an average of the findings among men and women. An alternative possibility, though, is that group membership is not a critical factor in and of itself but becomes important when other social ties are missing. The notions that individuals make trade-offs or substitutions in social relationships, and that mounting social isolation has greater disease consequences than the absence of any particular kind of contact, are supported by data presented in Chapter 4.

References

Belloc NB, Breslow L, Hochstim JR: Measurement of physical health in a general population survey. *Am. J. Epidemiol.* **93**(5):328–336, 1971.

Berkman LF: Social networks, host resistance, and mortality: a follow-up study of Alameda County Residents. Unpublished doctoral dissertation, University of California, Berkeley, Calif., 1977.

Berkman LF, Syme SL: Social networks, host resistance, and mortality: A nine-year follow-up study of Alameda County residents. *Am. J. Epidemiol.* **109**(2):186–204, 1979.

Brand RJ, Sholtz RI: A multiple adjustment method for combining J × 2 contingency tables for prospective and survival study analysis, paper presented at Biometrics Society Meeting, March 25, 1976.

Cahalan D, Cisin IH: American drinking practices: summary of findings from a national probability sample. II. Measurement of massed versus spaced drinking. *Q. J. Studies Alcohol* **29**:642–656, 1968.

Cahalan D, Cisin IH, Crossley HM: *American drinking practices: national study of drinking behavior and attitudes* New Brunswick: Rutgers Center of Alcohol Studies, 1969.

Hudes M: *Improvements in Screening Effectiveness and Efficiency from Increasing the Number of Predictors in Logistic Analysis*, Ph.D. dissertation, University of California, Berkeley, 1980.

Mantel N, Haenszel W: Statistical aspects of the analysis of data from retrospective studies of disease. *J. Natl. Cancer Inst.* **22**:719–748, 1959.

Rosenman RH, Brand RJ, Sholtz RI, et al.: Multivariate prediction of coronary heart disease during 8.5 year follow-up in the Western Collaborative Group Study. *Am. J. Cardiol.* **37**:903–910, 1976.

Truett J, Cornfield J, Kannel W: A multivariate analysis of the risk of coronary heart disease in Framingham. *J. Chron. Dis.* **20**:511–524, 1967.

Walker SH, Duncan DB: Estimation of the probability of an event as a function of several variables. *Biometrika* **54**:167–179, 1967.

6. Health practices, social networks, and change in physical health

TERRY C. CAMACHO   JAMES A. WILEY

Introduction

The preceding chapters of this volume have shown that certain aspects of our way of living are clearly and significantly associated with our risk of death. The findings presented are consistent with the idea that poor health, and resultant mortality risk, is a function of susceptibility to disease in general, as well as of disease-specific causal agents. It also appears that factors in the personal and social environments influence this susceptibility. In this chapter we will consider whether the same social conditions and behaviors that correlate with subsequent mortality risk, namely health practices and social ties, also predict variations in subsequent health status.

Because death is generally regarded as the end point of the spectrum along which health is measured—as the final stage of the disease process —deteriorating health status may be viewed as an earlier stage along that same spectrum. Given this perspective, one might question the usefulness of repeating the analysis of health practices and social networks on health using an outcome measure somewhere along, rather than at the end of the same spectrum. This objection would perhaps be valid if serious disease always resulted in death and did so in a predictable period of time. The fact is, however, that the health threats we face today are mainly the chronic diseases, which may continue with little change for many years, resulting in death only after a very long time, if at all. Risk of death from the biggest killers of today—heart disease, cancer, and cerebrovascular disease—includes at least two components: the risk of getting an illness (incidence) and the risk of dying from that illness (survival time). Mortality rates, of necessity, include both components. Using a simple analysis of mortality, it is usually not possible to distinguish whether one or the other, or both of these components, are responsible for correlations with other variables.

In the present volume, this problem has been dealt with partially by analyzing mortality rates while controlling for 1965 health status (Chapters 3 and 4). In this way, a separate relationship between the "survival component" and health practices and social network variables was demonstrated. In this chapter we will address the other part of the issue by analyzing morbidity outcomes among survivors of the panel sample. We will examine 1974 health status in relation to 1965 health practices and social networks in order to ascertain whether declining health status also varies with these factors. By using a broadly defined measure of health status, we will again examine the idea that disease states in general have some common antecedents.

Our interest in identifying any associations of health practices and social ties with health status separately from their relationships to mortality risk associated with disease is more than theoretical, however. Although many chronic illnesses may not result in death, or only after a very long time, most do result in some sort of disability or pain, or both. The personal, social, and economic losses associated with long-term chronic illness or impairment are enormous. Our ability to lengthen life today is remarkable, but the more years we are able to add to an individual's life span, the more we must be concerned about the level of well-being the individual experiences during those extra years. Thus it is critically important that we understand the factors that add or detract from one's overall ability to function fully in the physical realm, regardless of whether they also lengthen life.

Significance of the panel analysis

As noted in Chapter 3, previous HPL research has established a link between health practices and health status on a cross-sectional basis (Belloc and Breslow, 1972). This link is confirmed in a number of other studies (Chafetz et al., 1974; Palmore, 1971; Pesznecker and McNeil, 1975). Such cross-sectional findings, however, do not allow us to draw conclusions about the causal order of the variables. In fact, there is reason to suspect that at least part of the association between such practices as exercise, height/weight ratios, or sleeping habits and concurrent health status results from the effects of poor health on these factors rather than the reverse.

To date, longitudinal studies of health and health practices in which this problem of reverse causation could be controlled or eliminated have been few. Most of those that have been reported suffer from the limitation of small sample size, or they have been carried out with special groups selected on the basis of characteristics such as age or availability. Such studies do not permit generalization to a larger population. Also, although earlier chapters of this volume have shown clearly the longitudinal relationship of social networks and health practices to mortality, the question regarding the relationships of these items to the future health of survivors has not been addressed. The analysis presented here overcomes a number of these difficulties. It uses a large sample drawn from a general non-institutional population of adults, measuring social networks, health practices, and health status variables at two points in time 9 years apart.

An overview of the chapter

As indicated above, the analysis reported here differs from those in other chapters. It focuses on the *survivors* of the 1965 sample and their subsequent (1974) health status. A few words are therefore in order at this point regarding the methods used and the relationship of the findings to other HPL work in this volume and elsewhere.

First, it should be recognized that among the cohort being examined, changes in health will have occurred over the 9 years between 1965 and 1974. Generally, the changes will have been negative simply as a result of the aging process. Physical health status tends to deteriorate with age. Our interest lies in identifying departures—in either direction—from this expected change in health, and in examining the association of these deviations with configurations of health practices and social network factors.

The quantitative approach used for this task is a rather highly technical one because health status, and especially change in health status, is a complex concept that is difficult to quantify. We also make use of some relatively sophisticated statistical techniques, including certain regression procedures, to deal with the possibility of competing explanations for observed changes in health status. With these techniques we are able to examine changes in health status between 1965 and 1974, for given levels of initial health and for different age-sex groups, and then to measure the direction and extent of any deviation from the change expected on the basis of original health status and age and sex.

Although the development of this "residual health change score" is somewhat complex, the measure itself has a relatively straightforward meaning: negative values signify an excessive decline in health status (and associated risk of death) over that which would be expected given the individual's age, sex, and initial health; whereas positive values characterize individuals whose health has declined less than expected (and perhaps improved) over the 9-year period. A score of zero indicates that the observed change in health was the same as what was expected.

Whereas health outcome is thus measured differently here than in the mortality studies, and the methodology used varies from previous work, the basic results of our analysis confirm earlier cross-sectional findings regarding health practices and health status (Belloc and Breslow, 1972), and are entirely consistent with the mortality findings presented in this volume and elsewhere (Belloc, 1973). That is, using somewhat different methods and a subset of the original sample, we still find strong evidence to support the hypothesis that the health practices people follow and their social ties have significant impacts on their physical health.

There is one respect in which our findings appear to be inconsistent with earlier HPL findings, and that is in regard to the roles of breakfast and snacking as health practices. Previous work has shown eating breakfast regularly and abstaining from between-meal snacks to be associated with better than average health (Belloc, 1973; Belloc and Breslow, 1972); however, we have excluded these two items from this analysis because neither was a significant predictor of variations in health change between 1965 and 1974. This inconsistency may very well be ascribable to differences described above in methodology or to the fact that our sample is only a portion of the original 1965 survey sample.

The next section of this chapter will describe the sample, the data, and the method used in this analysis. The issue of panel loss will be addressed. In the section after that we will present our findings in three major parts: (1) the relationship of 1965 health practices to 1974 health status; (2) the relationship of 1965 social networks to 1974 health status; and (3) the joint contribution of health practices and social networks to subsequent health status. The first two will each include tests for measurement error and for possible confounding by the relationship of the variables to socioeconomic status.

Data and methods

The sample

The 1965-1974 panel sample has been described in detail in Chapter 2. For this analysis we use a subset of the panel sample consisting only of those members who were under 70 years of age in 1965 and of majority (white) ethnic status. The age limitation was based on the principle that risk factors such as health habits and social ties tend to lose predictive ability in advanced age. Preliminary analysis of our sample, which shows nonsignificant associations between health practices in 1965 and subsequent change in health status for persons over 70, was consistent with this possibility. Nonwhites were excluded from the analysis to avoid confounding with known correlations among race, health status, and lifestyle. The resulting sample, then, consists of 3892 white adults who were between 16 and 70 years of age in 1965 and for whom we have information on health and behaviors from questionnaires returned in 1965 and in 1974. It should be kept in mind that this sample differs somewhat from the sample used for the mortality analysis in earlier chapters of this volume.

Panel loss

The problem of bias resulting from panel attrition is by its very nature not amenable to complete solution. In any large community sample, some respondents will be lost to follow-up because of death, refusal, or inability to locate them. Hence there will always be a degree of uncertainty regarding the way in which the missing information might have changed the results of the analysis. The best that can be done in this situation is to estimate the likelihood of serious bias on the basis of what is known about the differences or similarities between those respondents who were retained in the study and those who were not.

Table 6-1 shows the panel attrition among the baseline respondents constituting the subset chosen for this analysis. Because we are investi-

Table 6-1. Distribution of white persons under 70 years of age in 1965 who returned a 1965 survey questionnaire according to status in 1974 follow-up study

Follow-up status	Number of cases	Percentage
Returned 1974 questionnaire ("panel members")	3892	76.2
Not located in 1974 follow-up	334 ⎫	6.5 ⎫
	⎬ 923	⎬ 18.0
Known survivor, failed to return 1974 questionnaire[a] ("dropouts")	589 ⎭	11.5 ⎭
Died 1965–1974	293	5.7

[a]This category consists primarily of refusals and cases in which follow-up after questionnaire placement was impossible or failed to yield results. It includes also a few cases in which the respondents were unable to complete the questionnaire as a result of senility or language problems, or in which an unusable questionnaire was returned.

gating the ability of health practices and social networks to predict future health status among survivors, we are not concerned with the 6 percent loss from known deaths. Among those who were not known to have died by 1974, the follow-up success rate in the younger, white subset used for this analysis is slightly higher than in the sample as a whole: 81 percent as compared to 78 percent. Nevertheless, if the 923 dropouts differ significantly from the 3892 panel members studied, our results could be seriously biased.

Table 6-2 provides a comparison of panel members and dropouts with respect to demographic characteristics and the variables used in this analysis. The dropout group includes a somewhat higher proportion of men and of younger persons than does the panel member group. The dropouts are also more apt to be in the lower income categories and to have somewhat fewer years of schooling. The two groups are nearly identical in terms of our measure of baseline health status; however, the dropouts show a tendency to have slightly lower scores on both the Health Practices Index and the Social Network Index.

The differences in demographic and other relevant characteristics are small but should be kept in mind in generalizing our findings to other populations. However, these differences in marginal distributions are not necessarily a source of bias affecting the hypotheses being considered here. The issue is whether our estimates of the *relation* between health practices and subsequent health status, or between social networks and subsequent health status, will be biased by analyzing only panel member data. The question, therefore, is whether there is reason to believe that the relationships between the social and behavioral variables and future health in the dropout group differ significantly from those we are measuring in the panel member group.

The method we have chosen to assess this kind of bias consists of comparing the relationships of health practices and social networks to health in each group at baseline and establishing a rationale for assuming some continuity between these cross-sectional relationships and the corresponding longitudinal relationships. If the two groups are similar in their baseline relationships, and if we can observe continuity between the cross-sectional and longitudinal relationships among the panel member group, then we will assume that the missing longitudinal relationship among dropouts would have been similar to that observed in this analysis and that we do not have significant or systematic bias.

Table 6-3 shows the health practices–health status relationships for panel members and dropouts at baseline. The overall direction and magnitude of the relationships are clearly the same for both groups, even

Table 6-2. Comparisons between panel members and dropouts with respect to sex, age, income, physical health status, and health practices score in 1965

Characteristic	Percentage of panel members (N = 3892)	Percentage of dropouts (N = 923)
1. Sex		
Male	45.0	48.5
Female	55.0	51.5
	100.0	100.0
2. Age in 1965 (years)		
16–33	35.1	43.2
34–51	42.6	37.9
52–69	22.3	18.8
	100.0	99.9
3. Family income level in 1965[a]		
Inadequate	6.7	9.9
Marginal	11.9	19.1
Adequate	48.8	49.0
Very adequate	32.5	22.0
	99.9	100.0
4. Years of schooling[b]		
0–8	9.3	13.3
9–11	15.0	23.9
12	34.5	31.3
13 or more	41.1	31.4
	99.9	99.9
5. Physical health status score in 1965[c]		
1–2, Disabled	10.2	11.5
3–4, ≥ 1 Chronic conditions	27.0	25.9
5, ≥ 1 Symptom	32.2	32.1
6–7, No symptoms	30.5	30.6
	99.9	100.1
6. Health practices score in 1965		
1	2.0	3.3
2	11.1	15.3
3	30.2	30.9
4	39.2	36.9
5	17.6	13.5
	100.1	99.9
7. Social Network Index		
Low	8.4	13.9
Medium	32.2	36.8
Medium-high	28.7	24.5
High	30.8	24.8
	100.1	100.0

[a]Because of missing data on income, these percentages are based on $N = 3774$ for panel members and $N = 858$ for dropouts. This income measure adjusts total family income by the number of persons in the household to establish adequacy of income level. For a family of three or four an annual income of $10,000 or more in 1965 is considered very adequate; between $5000 and $9999 is adequate; $3000–$4999 is labeled marginal; and below $3000 is considered inadequate.
[b]Because of missing data on years of schooling, these percentages are based on $N = 3881$ for panel members and $N = 919$ for dropouts.
[c]This score is described in detail in Belloc et al. (1971).

Table 6-3. Comparison between panel members and dropouts with respect to percentage distribution of physical health status in 1965 by 1965 health practices score

Health Practices Index summary score, 1965	Physical Health Status Index category, 1965			Total	N
	1–3	4–5	6–7		
0–1					
Panel	33.3	50.7	16.0	100.0	75
Dropouts	35.5	45.2	19.4	100.1	31
2					
Panel	24.1	52.0	23.9	100.0	431
Dropouts	26.2	53.2	20.6	100.0	141
3					
Panel	20.1	52.5	27.5	100.1	1176
Dropouts	18.3	53.0	28.8	100.1	285
4					
Panel	15.1	53.1	31.8	100.0	1526
Dropouts	17.0	48.1	34.9	100.0	341
5					
Panel	12.0	49.3	38.7	100.0	684
Dropouts	13.6	49.6	36.8	100.0	125

though there are minor variations in some cells. Similarly, Table 6-4 shows that the cross-sectional relationship of social network scores and health status scores is much the same for dropouts as for panel members. Only among those with the lowest social network scores are there sizeable differences between the two groups, and this difference is that a smaller percentage of dropouts than panel members show a low network–positive health combination—a combination that is infrequent in the main findings of this analysis. Thus if the dropouts had been included in this analysis, and the longitudinal relationship had corresponded to this cross-sectional one, this difference would only have strengthened the results obtained with the panel members actually studied.

There is reason to assume an overall continuity between the cross-sectional relationships and the longitudinal relationships of social networks and health practices to health status. First, because causation most likely works both ways (i.e., low-risk behaviors producing good health and good health predisposing toward low-risk behaviors), some stability in the relationship is built in. Second, to the extent that the health habits and social networks are relatively stable, the cross-sectional relationships may in fact also reflect longitudinal relationships; that is, social and behavioral characteristics measured in 1965 may also represent those

Table 6-4. Comparison between panel members and dropouts with respect to percentage distribution of physical health status in 1965 by 1965 Social Network Index scores

Social Network Index score, 1965	Physical Health Status Index category, 1965			Total	N
	1–3	4–5	6–7		
Low					
Panel	19.1	51.7	29.2	100.0	325
Dropouts	18.0	60.2	21.9	100.1	128
Medium					
Panel	17.5	51.1	31.4	100.0	1254
Dropouts	20.0	48.8	31.2	100.0	340
Medium-high					
Panel	16.2	55.0	28.8	100.0	1116
Dropouts	18.6	50.0	31.4	100.0	226
High					
Panel	18.1	50.4	31.6	100.1	1197
Dropouts	18.3	48.0	33.6	99.9	229

characteristics as they had been for several years before 1965 and would continue to be. A comparison of the cross-sectional and longitudinal health status–health practices relationships in the panel sample does in fact show a high degree of continuity from one relationship to the other. We have no reason to think this would have been less true for the dropouts.

Measurement of health status

One of the early tasks of the HPL was the development of a health status measure adequate to its very broad generic concept of health. The measure developed is known as the Physical Health Status Index, and it has been used in a number of earlier HPL publications as well as earlier chapters of this volume (Belloc et al., 1971). Its development is described in detail in Chapter 2. This measure takes into account functional level as well as presence or absence of specific disease states and symptoms. Respondents are scored from (1) to (7) according to the most serious health problem they report, as follows: (1) severe disability (has trouble feeding self, dressing, moving around, climbing stairs, or is unable to work); (2) less disability (had to change work or cut down, stop or cut down other activities); (3) two or more chronic conditions or impairments reported;

(4) one chronic condition reported; (5) one or more symptoms reported; (6) free of symptoms with low or medium energy level; and (7) free of symptoms with higher than average energy level.

This measure of health status met our criteria for a broad generic definition of health. In addition, using it allowed direct comparisons of our analysis with earlier HPL work in which this measure was used. However, choice of this index also presented some problems. The measure is an ordinal measure at best. The natural number scoring, from (1) to (7), creates an artificially even metric from one category to the next; we know this does not represent the actual magnitude of each successive step of the index in terms of any associated risk.

The solution to this problem seemed to be to retain the index categories as defined and to divide the sample into health status groups on this basis, but to find a way to assign meaningful quantitative values to these categories. We chose to quantify the Health Status Index in terms of mortality risk as the most logical and reliable quantitative measure available to us. To do this we used 9-year age-standardized survival rates from the original 1965 HPL sample ($N = 6928$), and substituted the survival rates associated with each Health Status Index category in that sample for the original number scores of the index. This rescaling of the Physical Health Status Index scores was then applied to our sample for both the 1965 and 1974 measurements of health status. In this way, we retained the designation of functional ability and of presence or absence of disease in our index *categories*, but assigned numerical values to those categories that represent risk more accurately than the natural number scores and allow us to use analytical tools appropriate for data measured on an interval or ratio scale.

Table 6-5 shows the recoded values corresponding to each original value of the Physical Health Status Index. The rescaled scores are, as predicted, strikingly nonlinear. The distance between categories measured in terms of associated survivorship decreases sharply as one moves from low to high levels of health, indicating that the upper end of the index discriminates more finely between degrees of mortality risk than does the lower end. To put it another way, a difference in health status between, for example, severe and moderate disability (original scores 1 and 2) has much greater significance in terms of risk of death than does a difference between, for example, one chronic condition and symptoms only (original scores 4 and 5).

Table 6-5 also shows the distribution of our panel sample on the 1965 measure of physical health. This distribution is obviously skewed toward the healthier end of the spectrum, with about 63 percent of the respondents

Table 6-5. Scoring of the Physical Health Status Index categories

Physical Health Status Index categories[a]	Age-standardized survival rates[b] (per 100)	Distribution of panel sample by health status score
1	77.0	126
2	88.0	271
3	90.8	281
4	91.8	771
5	92.5	1255
6, 7	93.2	1188
Total		3892

[a]Belloc et al. (1971).
[b]The standardized rate S_J for the Jth health status category was calculated in the following way:

$$S_J = 100 - \sum_I \frac{D_{IJ}N_I}{N_{IJ}N} 100$$

where D_{IJ} = number of deaths 1965–1974 of persons in the Ith age group and Jth health status category in 1965; N_{IJ} = number of persons at risk in the Ith age group and the Jth health status category in 1965; $N_I = \sum_J N_{IJ}$; and $N = \sum_I N_I = 6928$.

Three age groups were used to standardize the rates: 16–44, 45–64, and 65–99 years.

in the three highest health status categories. This is partly a result of the fact that we have selected for our sample only those who were under 70 in 1965, white, and who survived at least until 1974.

Table 6-6 shows the changes in the panel respondents' average physical health status scores between 1965 and 1974 by age, sex, and a rough measure of health practices. (A finer version of this measure is described in the next main section, under Findings.) All age-sex groups in the sample experience a decline in average health status scores over the 9-year period. As expected, the magnitude of this decline increases with advancing age for both men and women. Further, this trend characterizes both low-risk and high-risk groups. Those with low-risk (i.e., more favorable) health practices show a smaller decline in health status score than the high-risk group. The difference is consistent through all age and sex groups, and it is substantially greater among persons over 45 years of age. This finding anticipates the results reported in greater detail later in this chapter, namely that the advantage in 1974 of those who maintain low-risk health practices over those who practice few is not simply a function of their more favorable health status in 1965; rather it reflects a real difference between the two groups in the degree of change in health status over time. The methodology described below will be used to investigate this difference more carefully by examining individual deviations from expected changes in health status within categories of age, sex, and initial health.

Table 6-6. Mean rescaled Physical Health Status scores, 1965 and 1974, by age, sex, and health practices score

	Total sample		Low health practices score (0–3)		High health practices score (4–5)	
Sex and age (years) 1965	1965	1974	1965	1974	1965	1974
Male (total)	91.9	90.9	91.6	90.2	92.1	91.3
16–29	92.5	92.0	92.4	91.7	92.5	92.2
30–44	92.1	91.4	91.8	90.9	92.3	91.7
45–59	91.5	90.0	91.1	88.6	91.7	90.8
60–69	90.6	88.5	90.1	87.9	90.9	88.9
Female (total)	91.4	90.1	90.7	88.9	91.9	90.9
16–29	92.4	91.6	92.2	91.1	92.4	91.8
30–44	91.7	90.6	91.2	89.6	92.0	91.3
45–59	90.8	89.1	90.0	88.0	91.5	89.9
60–69	89.7	87.4	88.9	86.3	90.6	88.5

Methodology

In assessing the relationship of baseline health practices and social networks to subsequent health status, some obvious sources of possible confounding must be considered. Perhaps the most significant is initial health status. Previous chapters have shown that baseline health status and baseline health practices are correlated, and noted the possibility that health helps to determine, or at least to limit, health practices. Whereas physical health status, as measured by our index, is only moderately stable over the 9-year period (Pearson correlation = .48 between 1965 and 1974 measures), we can nevertheless say that about 25 percent of the variance in 1974 health status is "explained" by the 1965 health status score, whether through the mechanisms of health practices and social networks, associations with age, or heritable differences in susceptibility to illness. Also, there are significant age and sex differences in health status, health practices, and social networks, any of which could confound the relationships of the social and behavioral items to future health as they appear in our data.

Although a number of other possible sources of confounding could be listed (and indeed we will examine some of these later in this chapter), age, sex, and initial health were considered to be three fundamental and known sources that should be controlled at the outset. We therefore chose a methodology that allowed us to build controls for these three variables into our outcome measure (1974 health) so that the analysis could be done

in a fairly simple, straightforward manner without resorting to sophisticated multivariate techniques, but with adequate controls for these variables. This was accomplished with the following procedure:

1. The sample was divided into 12 age-sex groups using six 9-year age
   groups for each sex. The 9-year groupings were chosen to correspond
   to the period between measurements to create a "synthetic cohort."
2. For each of the 12 groups, using regression methods, we fitted a linear
   equation stating that health status in 1974 is a linear function of 1965
   health status scores.
3. The regression coefficients obtained in step 2 were used to calculate a
   predicted 1974 health status score for each age-sex group as follows:

$$\hat{H}(74) = a_i + b_i H(65)$$

Thus $\hat{H}(74)$ is the health status score we would "predict" for an
individual on the basis of what we know about the relationship of
initial health status to 1974 health status for individuals of that person's
age and sex.

4. The predicted value calculated in step 3 was then subtracted from the
   actual observed value of the 1974 physical health status for the individual, resulting in a "*residual*" 1974 health status score indicating how
   the individual's score *differs* from what was expected on the basis of
   age, sex, and initial health status.

The outcome health measure resulting from these steps, then, reflects
the extent to which respondents' 1974 health status scores exceeded or fell
short of their predicted scores for 1974. It is a measure of deviation, up or
down, from an expected score, and does not represent an absolute value
of health or survivorship status.

To illustrate, a residual health score of 0 would indicate that the
individual's 1974 health status score was the same as that which was
predicted for that person on the basis of sex, age in 1965, and initial health
status. An adjusted health score of —4, on the other hand, can be interpreted
as a survivorship/health status, which is 4 per 100 lower (less healthy) than
would be expected, given the individual's sex, age, and initial health
status, and a score of +4 indicates that the individual's status is 4 per 100
higher (healthier) than expected.

Residual health status scores in our sample range from −15.2 to +14.7.
More than one third of the sample score within one point of the predicted
score (−1 to +1), and nearly 70 percent within two points either side of
zero. Three fourths of the sample score better than predicted, but three
fourths of those are within one point of the predicted value, and only 3
percent of the sample exceeds their predicted scores by four points or
more toward the healthy end of the spectrum. Of those whose actual

follow-up health status was worse than predicted—that is, those with negative residual health scores (24% of the sample)—a little more than one third are one point or less below predicted values, and half are within two points, whereas 7.6 percent of the total sample are more than four points lower than expected.

Findings

Health practices and subsequent health status

In Chapter 3 data showing the association of mortality risk with each of the seven health practices were presented. These items (cigarette smoking, alcohol consumption, hours of sleep per night, exercise, height/weight ratio, and breakfast and snacking habits) were chosen on the basis of earlier HPL work that had shown them to be related to concurrent health status and to 5-year mortality.

In the 9-year mortality analysis, only five of the original seven habits were significantly associated with the risk of death; eating breakfast regularly and eating between meals showed unclear or weak relationships with mortality over the 9-year period, and the relationships did not reach statistical significance. The summary index used in the mortality analysis was thus constructed using only the first five of the health practices listed above.

Our preliminary analyses of the longitudinal data indicated a similar lack of relation between eating habits and residual health scores. Because of these findings, we present here no further analyses of the effects of regular breakfasts or snacking. As noted above, however, our failure to find significant associations between these factors and indices of physical health may result from conditions other than a lack of causal connection. Both the sample we used (whites only, 70 years and younger) and our method of analysis (comparing groups with respect to residual health scores) are quite different from those used in the earlier reports that showed health benefits from regular breakfasts and avoidance of snacks. Furthermore, use of more sensitive measures of diet and nutritional adequacy might very well generate findings that would lead us to include breakfast and not eating between meals in a list of "healthy behaviors."

In this section we will first examine the relationship of each of the five health practice items to health as measured by our residual health score. We will then assess the effects of multiple low- or high-risk health habits on health status using the same summary Index of Health Practices employed in the mortality analysis (Chapter 3). Data for these analyses are presented in Table 6-7. For each category of the individual health practices and for each score of the Health Practices Index, we present the mean

Table 6-7. Mean residual physical health score by 1965 cigarette consumption, alcohol consumption, hours of sleep, physical activity, obesity, and an Index of Health Practices

Health practices	Males				Females				Total			
	Mean residual	N	F-Ratio	P	Mean residual	N	F-Ratio	P	Mean residual	N	F-Ratio	P
1. Cigarette smoking, 1965			4.17	.000			.88	.513			3.94	.001
Never smoked	.29	531			.08	936			.16	1467		
Past smoker, ≤ 10/day	.64	97			.24	158			.39	255		
Past smoker, 20/day	.54	159			.42	75			.50	234		
Past smoker, ≥ 30/day	.02	138			−.26	44			−.05	182		
Current smoker, ≤ 10/day	.07	172			.12	290			.10	471		
Current smoker, 20/day	−.48	327			−.32	375			−.39	702		
Current smoker, ≥ 30/day	−.54	318			−.22	232			−.41	550		
2. Alcohol consumption (number of drinks per month), 1965[a]			2.05	.069			1.02	.403			2.58	.025
Nondrinker	−.61	199			−.35	407			−.44	606		
1–8 drinks/month	−.03	200			.08	507			.05	707		
9–16 drinks/month	−.07	320			.09	493			.03	813		
17–30 drinks/month	.27	441			.21	406			.24	847		
31–45 drinks/month	.30	185			.09	139			.21	324		
46 or more drinks/month	−.06	406			−.19	189			−.10	595		
3. Hours of sleep per day, 1965			2.80	.039			6.11	.000			7.57	.000
< 7 hrs/day	−.37	215			−.93	257			−1.66	126		
7 hrs/day	−.14	793			.13	819			−.00	1612		
8 hrs/day	.30	647			.22	881			.25	1528		
> 8 hrs/day	−.06	92			−.34	181			−.25	273		
4a. Leisure-time physical activity score, 1965[b]			3.21	.002			3.42	.001			6.06	.000
Total sample												
0 (Inactive)	−1.78	36			−1.61	90			−1.66	126		
1–2	−.45	139			−.56	248			−.52	387		
3–4	−.60	215			−.07	373			−.26	588		
5–6	.12	303			.25	446			.20	749		
7–8	.21	422			.15	475			.18	897		

	Mean	N	Mean	N	Mean	N	F		F		F	
9–10	.17	328	.25	291	.21	619						
11–12	.30	191	.16	154	.24	345						
13–16 (Very active)	.14	117	.51	64	.27	181						
4b. Leisure-time physical activity score, 1965, nondisabled only (N = 3495)							1.20	.053	3.60	.001	5.27	.000
0 (Inactive)	−.96	30	−1.88	62	−1.58	92						
1–2	−.58	112	−.67	201	−.64	313						
3–4	−.51	187	−.10	321	−.25	508						
5–6	.06	274	.04	398	.05	672						
7–8	.10	389	.23	442	.17	831						
9–10	.25	313	.16	273	.21	586						
11–12	.11	176	.20	142	.15	318						
13–16 (Very active)	.22	115	.43	60	.29	175						
5. Percent deviation from ideal weight for height, 1965[c]							3.80	.010	2.63	.049	5.51	.000
11% or more underweight	−.32	69	−.41	136	−.38	205						
±10% Ideal weight	.11	762	.20	1144	.16	1906						
11–29% Overweight	.06	771	−.07	595	.00	1366						
30% or more overweight	−.93	136	−.47	266	−.63	402						
6. Index of Health Practices							6.24	.000	6.60	.000	12.61	.000
0–1	−1.57	38	−1.63	37	−1.60	75						
2	−.65	199	−.74	232	−.70	431						
3	−.20	557	.28	619	−.24	1176						
4	.27	665	.22	861	.25	1526						
5	.41	292	.54	392	.48	684						

[a]Respondents reported frequency of drinking (number of times per week) and amount consumed (usual number of drinks per sitting) separately for beer, wine, and liquor. The monthly alcohol consumption score was derived by multiplying amount by frequency for each beverage category and summing these three products.

[b]Respondents were asked whether they often, sometimes, or never participated in each of the following: swimming or long walks, active sports, doing physical exercises, working in the garden, hunting, or fishing. Points were assigned for each activity according to the frequency of participation reported and the presumed strenuousness of the activity, with swimming, physical exercises, and active sports receiving twice the value of hunting/fishing and gardening. Points were summed across the five activity categories to obtain the total leisure-time physical activity score.

[c]Quetelet Index scores were derived using the formula: (weight in pounds/height in inches)^2. Using data on mean weights for medium-frame persons in each of eight height categories (from Metropolitan Life Insurance Co.), the Quetelet Index scores for 10% underweight, 10% overweight, and 30% overweight were calculated for each height category (separately for men and women). The mean of the scores for all categories was used to define the bound of the code categories used here. This index is used because it has been demonstrated that it accurately brings together people with the same proportionate weights.

residual health score values and the number of cases in that category. The significance of each association is assessed using one-way analysis of variance, and the F-ratios and their associated probability values are shown. Next, we test for the possibility of spurious or exaggerated findings caused by response errors. Finally, the relationship of health practices and health status, controlling for income and education, is examined as a means of checking for the possibility that socioeconomic status is a confounding variable in this relationship (Table 6-8).

CIGARETTE SMOKING

As expected, nonsmokers have better health status scores at follow-up than do those who were smoking in 1965. However, former smokers who smoked no more than 30 cigarettes a day have even higher adjusted health status scores than those who never smoked. Because the adjusted score is in fact a measure of change in health, this result is perhaps not surprising. Compared to persons who continue to smoke, former light or moderate smokers may indeed experience fewer symptoms or conditions, an increase in energy level, or both as a result of giving up cigarettes.

Number of cigarettes smoked daily is an important factor in the health of both former and current smokers. Those who were smoking less than one-half pack per day in 1965 had more favorable adjusted health scores in 1974 than did those who had quit smoking in 1965 but reported heavy smoking before that time. Again, it may be that some of these former heavy smokers started smoking again between 1965 and 1974, or that they had smoked for a greater number of years than the current light smokers. On the other hand, it is possible that the effects of heavy habitual smoking are still evident in health status 9 years or more after giving up the habit.

The impact of smoking habits on subsequent health is far more significant for men than for women in our sample, just as it was for mortality. For women, the association between smoking and subsequent physical health status is far from statistically significant. Further, there are some minor inconsistencies in the pattern of association between number of cigarettes and health for women. For example, both current and past smokers who smoke 30 or more per day seem to have more favorable adjusted health scores than those who smoke only 20 per day, although less favorable than the very lightest smokers. Until rather recently, far fewer women than men have been smokers, and these figures may therefore reflect shorter or less consistent smoking habits for women. It is also possible that smoking for women is linked with a different set of circumstances or other behaviors than it is for men, and that the relationship for one or both sexes is confounded by these other associated variables. For men, the association of health with amount smoked and recency of smoking is like that described for the total sample. Most former male smokers show a health change advantage over those who have never smoked.

ALCOHOL CONSUMPTION

Moderate consumption of alcohol (17–45 drinks per month) is associated in our sample with the most favorable trend in adjusted health scores for each sex and for the sample as a whole, conforming to the mortality findings. For women the pattern of association between alcohol consumption and subsequent health is the same as for men but not statistically significant. Heavy drinkers suffer unfavorable health outcomes as measured by our adjusted score. However, those who report that they do not drink any alcoholic beverages have even more negative adjusted health scores than the heavy drinkers. These results are consistent with other studies that have shown total abstention from alcohol to be associated with less than optimal health (Chafetz et al., 1974). Our findings are similar to those from the mortality analysis in Chapter 3 except that when mortality is the outcome measure, nondrinkers constitute the middle risk group (higher risk than moderate drinkers but lower than heavy drinkers) rather than the highest risk group, as they do in this analysis.

Two commonly proposed explanations of this pattern are not supported in our data. The reverse causation theory—that the abstainers include a large number of persons who quit drinking because of ill health—is countered in these data by the fact that initial health status controls are built into our outcome measure. Similarly, our age controls undermine the hypothesis that generational differences in attitudes toward drinking make the nondrinking group the oldest and therefore most likely to experience declines in health.

SLEEP PATTERNS

A definite curvilinear relation exists between hours of sleep per night and subsequent health as measured by the adjusted score. It is clear that 7 or 8 hours per night are optimal for health status as they were for mortality risk; the norm of 8 hours is associated with the highest adjusted health scores for both sexes. Individuals who regularly get less sleep than this have the least favorable adjusted health scores. However, those who sleep more than the apparently optimal 8 hours also show lower follow-up health status scores than predicted (negative residual scores). The effects of either too little or too much sleep on residual health scores are greater for women than for men, although the relationship is statistically significant for both. These results follow the same pattern observed in the baseline cross-sectional relationship of sleep and health as well as that of mortality rates and sleep habits.

Poor health can be related to sleep habits in either direction: it can be a cause of difficulty in sleeping, thus resulting in fewer hours per night; or illness can necessitate more than the usual amount of sleep per night. Similarly, older individuals generally require fewer hours of sleep on a regular basis than do young or middle-aged persons. Possibly the relationship of poor health or mortality to less than 7 hours of sleep derives from this age factor. The panel analysis makes it possible to conclude, however, that sleep habits influence future health regardless of age and initial health, because both of these are controlled within the adjusted follow-up health status measure.

LEISURE-TIME PHYSICAL ACTIVITY

Mean adjusted health scores tend to be higher with amount of physical activity in 1965 for both men and women. The difference between those who report no activity at all and those who report even a little is especially marked. There are small inconsistencies in the trend among individuals at moderate or higher levels of activity when the sample is broken down into a large number of physical activity categories as in Table 6-7. When subjects are grouped more broadly into low, medium, and high activity levels, the gradient is steady. These findings are quite similar to those in the mortality analysis and in the cross-sectional analysis.

The potential for reverse causation of health and health habits is perhaps more obvious in the case of exercise than with any other health practice. Health may be viewed as a measure of *capacity* to engage in physical activity, and thus any relationship between the two variables could plausibly be interpreted as reflecting the effect of health on the rate of activity rather than an indication of the beneficial effects of such activity on health. The fact that the health measure used here has been adjusted for level of initial health casts doubt on this explanation of the findings. Nevertheless, in this case a more stringent test for such possible confounding is warranted. We repeated the analysis of health and activity, excluding from the sample all persons who reported any physical disability in 1965. Section 4b in Table 6-7 presents the findings of this analysis. For men, removal of the disabled from the sample narrows the spread of mean adjusted health scores over activity levels, but a clear and significant relationship between activity level and health score remains. For women, and for the two sexes combined, the findings with and without the disabled individuals are nearly identical; exclusion of the disabled actually enhances the significance of the relationship slightly. We conclude that initial health, acting as an enabling factor, does not account in any large measure for the observed relationship between level of physical activity and mean adjusted health score in 1974.

WEIGHT IN RELATION TO HEIGHT

Height/weight ratios, expressed in terms of percentage deviation from ideal weight for height, show an interesting curvilinear relationship with health status. The extreme overweight category (30% or more over desirable weight for height) is associated with the poorest follow-up health scores. The next highest risk category is 10 percent or more *underweight*; among women, health scores for this group are only slightly better than those for the extremely overweight group. Individuals within 10 percent of their optimum weight have the best adjusted health scores, whereas those who are 11 to 29 percent overweight are at a slightly greater risk, women more than men.

The same generally curvilinear pattern was seen in the cross-sectional analysis of health habits and health, and in the mortality analysis summarized in Chapter 3. Mortality risk was highest for those in the extreme underweight category—for men, nearly twice as high as for those who were 30 percent or more overweight. However, the excess risk associated with being underweight as opposed to being extremely overweight is not seen in this analysis of follow-up health status, where initial health status is controlled. This suggests that at least part of the reason for the very high mortality rates among underweight persons is that this group includes a number of people who have suffered weight loss from disease before their death. Numbers were too small in the mortality analysis to test this directly by stratifying the sample according to health status. On the basis of our panel data, it appears that whereas obesity is the greater health risk, being underweight may also contribute to poor health.

HEALTH PRACTICES INDEX

Combining all of the health habit practices into an index permits measuring health-relevant behaviors in a more general way than is possible with any single habit. The index is constructed by dichotomizing each of the five health practices and assigning one point for each item on which the respondent falls into the half of the dichotomy that is associated with more favorable health outcomes. (See Chapter 3 for a detailed description of the construction of this index and of cutpoints used in establishing the dichotomies.) Thus scores on the index correspond to the number of low-risk health practices that an individual follows.

Table 6-7 shows the mean follow-up health scores associated with each Health Practices Index category. Because the items were dichotomized for use in the index, some of the fine discrimination possible with the full spread of the items is lost. Nevertheless, for the sample as a whole, the range of health scores over the index categories is greater than the range associated with any single health practice, and much greater than most. When compared to the discrimination obtained using individual health practices in their dichotomous index form, the power of the index is very clear: the range of scores is three times as great for the index as for any single health practice. This finding is important because it establishes that the individual health practice items are not redundant measures of the same factor; that is, to some extent at least, they represent independent factors that in combination have a greater impact than does any one alone.

The relationship of 1965 Health Practices Index scores to 1974 residual health status scores holds for men and for women separately. These findings are in conformity with the results of the mortality and health practices study discussed in Chapter 3, where it was found that the Index of Health Practices, even grouped into a trichotomous form, discriminated more effectively among mortality rates than did any of the individual practices. The panel analysis results presented in this chapter, by providing controls on initial health status, also lend validity to the findings in the cross-sectional analysis of health and health practices. The health habits are predictive of changes in health status over time.

MEASUREMENT ERROR

The health measure used in this study is based on self-reports of chronic conditions, symptoms, activity limitations, and energy level. These have been found to correlate fairly highly with information obtained from medical records and to be relatively stable over short periods of time (Graham, 1963; Hochstim et al., 1968). Nevertheless, some part of the variability in health scores undoubtedly results from response errors rather than from real variability in general health. Such errors ordinarily attenuate relationships between the fallible measure and a criterion. In the present study, however, because it uses residualized scores as outcome measures, such errors can create a bias that spuriously enhances the association between the criterion and other variables (Bereiter, 1967; Wiley and Camacho, 1980).

As a partial check on the effects of response errors, we recalculated mean adjusted health scores for each health practices summary score, assuming four different rates of error variance in the health status measure: 10, 20, 30, and 40 percent. We found that the positive association between

1965 health practices summary scores and subsequent mean adjusted health scores is not seriously affected by adjustment of the data for measurement error. For men, the mean values of the residual health score for each category of the Health Practices Index are nearly constant over the range from 10 to 40 percent in the amount of assumed measurement error. The F-ratios, though somewhat reduced at each successively higher level of assumed error, are still all significant at the .01 level or better. For women, the spread of the mean adjusted scores from the highest to the lowest index category is reduced by the corrections for measurement error, but the relationship remains significant at better than .03 level until the maximum of 40 percent error variance is assumed. We conclude from these results that measurement error is not a plausible alternative explanation for the findings presented thus far.

SOCIOECONOMIC STATUS, HEALTH PRACTICES, AND SUBSEQUENT HEALTH STATUS

Much evidence shows that persons of lower socioeconomic status (as defined by a number of measures) have higher morbidity, disability, and mortality rates than do those in the upper strata (Graham, 1963; Hochstim et al., 1968; National Center for Health Statistics, 1965; Syme and Berkman, 1976; "Socioeconomic Differentials," 1972). Also, some of the health practices considered in this analysis are more typical of high socioeconomic status groups than of low (Khosla and Lowe, 1972; U.S., D.H.E.W., 1973; "Socioeconomic Differentials," 1972). It is therefore possible that class-related "coping styles," including smoking, eating, and drinking habits, may be one of the mechanisms by which low socioeconomic status induces a generalized susceptibility to disease (Syme and Berkman, 1976). On the other hand, if the impact of socioeconomic status on health is primarily through mechanisms *other* than health habits, then the fact that both health and health practices are related to socioeconomic status could "explain away" the health practices–health status relationships found in this study.

The data in Table 6-8 shed some light on these issues for our sample. Section A of the table presents the interrelationships among adjusted health scores, health practices, and socioeconomic status as measured by income level (family income adjusted for family size). The relationship of health practices to health change scores persists at all income levels. The relationship between health habits and health change scores is strongest for low-income groups; similarly, the relationship between income and residual health scores is most dramatic among those with higher risk health practices. The gradients for both independent variables—health practices and income—are remarkably clear and consistent, with the entire gradient for one risk variable shifting up with each step of improve-

Table 6-8. Mean residual physical health score by Index of Health Practices controlling for income and years of schooling

A. Family income, health practices, and mean residual change scores

1965 Family income (adjusted for size of household)	Index of Health Practices, 1965									
	0–2		3		4		5		Total	
	Mean	N	Mean	N	Mean	N	Mean	N	Mean	N
Inadequate or marginal	−1.67	110	−.80	222	−.24	256	.38	115	−.54	703
Adequate	−.89	221	−.20	564	.19	738	.42	320	−.02	1843
Very adequate	−.09	161	.08	352	.68	487	.54	228	.38	1228

Analysis of variance summary	Sum of squares	DF	Mean square	F-Ratio	P
Main effects	973.62	5	194.72	13.793	.001
Family income	381.43	2	190.72	13.509	.001
Index of Health Practices, 1965	592.19	3	197.40	13.982	.001
Interaction of income and health practices	79.16	6	13.19	.935	.469
Residual	53111.44	3762	14.12		
Total	54164.22	3773	14.36		

B. Years of schooling, health practices, and mean residual change scores

Years of schooling completed in 1965	Index of Health Practices, 1965									
	0–2		3		4		5		Total	
	Mean	N	Mean	N	Mean	N	Mean	N	Mean	N
0–11	−1.25	155	−1.06	331	−.41	345	.19	115	−.71	946
12	−.84	185	−.04	388	.47	556	.59	210	.16	1336
13 or more	−.37	163	.16	452	.41	622	.51	359	.28	1596

Analysis of variance summary	Sum of squares	DF	Mean square	F-Ratio	P
Main effects	1160.81	5	232.16	16.370	.001
Years of schooling	626.68	2	313.34	22.094	.001
Index of Health Practices, 1965	534.13	3	178.04	12.554	.001
Interaction of schooling and health practices	72.49	6	12.08	.852	.530
Residual	54871.51	3869	14.18		
Total	56104.81	3880	14.46		

ment on the other risk factor. Overall, these data indicate that income level and health practices are additive in their impact on future health status. A two-way analysis of variance shows that both income and health habits are significant in their effects on health change scores $(P = .001)$, whereas the interaction effects of the two are not significant. In this analysis of variance we used a hierarchical method in which the effects of income were partialed out before examining the effects of health practices, in order to give the socioeconomic status variable the fullest possible chance to "explain away" the relationship between health practices and health status. Despite this conservative approach, the observed influence of health habits remains strong.

In Part B of Table 6-8, the analysis is repeated using education as the socioeconomic status risk variable. Education is perhaps a more reliable measure of socioeconomic status than income because, in an adult population, it is more likely than income to remain stable over time and, unlike income, it is relatively little affected by changes in health status. In these data the interrelationships among educational level, health practices, and adjusted health scores are much like those described above in which income was the socioeconomic measure. Residual 1974 health scores improve with higher health practices scores at all levels of education. Also, health scores generally improve as years of schooling increase, for all health practices score levels.

Overall, the data indicate additive influences on health status from education and health habits. Again, the analysis of variance shows that both schooling and health habits are significant at the .001 level of probability, whereas the interaction effects of these two variables on health status are non-significant. We conclude that the effects of health practices on future health cannot be accounted for by variation in income or in educational level. Neither can the importance of socioeconomic status to health be explained to any significant extent by class differences in health habits.

This analysis indicates that both kinds of factors, socioeconomic and health habits, make significant independent contributions to consequent health, and that as risk factors their influence is additive.

Social networks and subsequent health status

In Chapter 4 it was demonstrated that level of social involvement, as measured by an index of intimate and nonintimate ties with other people, was associated with different mortality risks. A number of previous studies were cited as demonstrating similar links between mortality, morale, and health status, both physical and psychological. In this section we will show that social network variables, and especially a summary index of various network ties, also predict subsequent health as measured by our adjusted health change score. Data in support of this are presented in Table 6-9.

MARITAL STATUS

Of the individual social network measures considered here, marital status is most strongly related to adjusted health scores for the sample as a whole. Among men, the married are in the most favorable position. Those who were never married have a slightly negative residual health score, whereas those who were formerly married—the separated, divorced, or widowed—are at greater risk in terms of future health. This is very much like the findings on mortality and marital status.

Among the women in our sample, however, a different pattern emerges, one unlike the mortality findings. The formerly married are again in the least favorable position. On the other hand, those who were never married have considerably better follow-up health scores than predicted, by a greater margin than the currently married.

A number of possible explanations come to mind for the fact that single unmarrieds of both sexes are so much better off than those who are unmarried by reason of separation, divorce, or widowhood. First, although the age control built into the adjusted health score measure is very strong, it is less than perfect. Some age effect may be occurring because the singles are generally quite young, and the widowed are primarily from the oldest part of the sample. It may also be that singleness relates to social networks very differently for the never married than for the formerly married. The latter group is likely to have built a network around the relationship with the spouse, mutually with other couples, in-laws' activities, and organizations that they enjoy together. Loss of the spouse may then disrupt this entire structure, leaving the individual relatively isolated unless new networks can be established. Those who have never married, on the other hand, are more likely to have built social networks based on their individual relationships. In many cases they may be living with a partner with whom a marriage-like relationship is maintained.

It is also possible that the relative disadvantage of married women as compared to singles is related to the health risks and stresses involved in parenthood. To test this notion we compared the married women who had never had children with those who had. We discovered that married women who have not borne children have a mean residual health score of .43 as compared to .06 for all married women, .00 for married women who have had children, and .69 for single (never married) women.

Table 6-9. Mean residual physical health score by marital status, friends and relatives index, group membership score, church group membership, and Social Network Index

Social network items	Males				Females				Total			
	Mean residual	N	F-Ratio	P	Mean residual	N	F-Ratio	P	Mean residual	N	F-Ratio	P
1. Marital status, 1965												
Never married	-.19	199	6.35	.002	.69	197	9.36	.000	.25	396	12.85	.000
Married	.09	1468			.06	1669			.08	3137		
Separated, divorced, or widowed	-1.25	84			-.86	275			-.95	359		
2. Friends and relatives index, 1965												
Low	-.53	239	3.28	.038	-.59	251	3.21	.041	-.56	490	6.33	.002
Medium	.09	1138			.11	1435			.10	2573		
High	.06	374			.01	455			.02	829		
3. Group memberships, 1965												
None	-.11	414	.580	.447	-.23	844	4.38	.037	-.19	1258	4.62	.032
One or more	.03	1337			.15	1297			.16	2634		
4. Church-group membership, 1965												
No	-.10	1305	4.51	.034	-.02	1527	.193	.661	-.06	2832	2.65	.104
Yes	.30	446			.06	614			.16	1060		
5. Social Network Index, 1965												
Low	-.66	118	3.12	.025	-.72	207	2.49	.059	-.70	325	4.86	.002
Medium	-.17	494			.02	760			-.06	1254		
Medium-high	-.01	575			.13	542			.06	1116		
High	.29	565			.11	632			.19	1197		

Clearly, there is a negative association between parity and the health change score here, although, once again, the age factor may account for some of it.

FRIENDS AND RELATIVES

The second item in Table 6-9 is the index of contacts with friends and relatives to whom an individual feels close. These ties, which represent a middle ground between the intimate relationship of spouse and the more formal affiliations with organized groups, discriminate rather clearly among our sample in terms of future health. For men and women alike, involvement with close friends and relatives (other than spouse) is associated with higher than expected health scores. For both men and women, low involvement is related to lower levels of health status in 1974. These findings essentially duplicate the findings in Chapter 4 relating mortality and contacts with friends and relatives.

ORGANIZATION MEMBERSHIP

More formal social ties, as measured by membership in organizations of various kinds and by church group membership, are related to subsequent adjusted health status in the expected direction for both sexes. Membership in one or more organizations (other than church group) is associated with a slightly more positive residual health status score than nonmembership, just as it was associated with a somewhat lower mortality rate overall. This relationship is statistically significant for women but not for men. Church-group membership is also associated with more positive follow-up health scores; but here the relationship is significant for men whereas it is not for women.

THE SOCIAL NETWORK INDEX

The results presented thus far comprise impressively consistent evidence that social ties have a significant impact on future health. Because our methodology controls for initial health status and for age, these results do not reflect only the loss of contacts and roles that can accompany either illness or old age. The last item in Table 6-9 is the Social Network Index, which combines all four of the previous items in a summary measure of network size. (See Chapters 2 and 4 for detailed description of how this index is constructed.) For both sexes the gradient of residual health scores over the four categories of the index is in the predicted direction. The spread of the mean health scores is greater over the range of social network scores than over the range of any single network item except marital status. The improvement in residual health scores with successively higher network scores is steady, except for women at the top two levels of the Social Network Index where the gradient levels off. For both sexes the biggest differences in health scores are found between the two lowest categories of the Social Network Index, suggesting that existence of some minimal level of social contact is a critical factor in health, whereas increased contacts beyond that provide somewhat smaller increments in protection against health risks. The pattern of association of Social Network Index scores with residual health change scores is much like that between social network scores and mortality rates.

MEASUREMENT ERROR

With the social network scores, as with the health practices scores, it is reasonable to examine the extent to which our results might be influenced by measurement error in the health status measure. Using the same approach as that described in the earlier section on findings (p. 196) regarding the relationship of health habits and residual health scores (Wiley and Camacho, 1980), we examined the mean values of residual health scores by social network scores for each of four assumed percentages of error variance. Overall, it may be said that the possibility of error variance represents a slightly more serious problem in the social network analysis than it did with health practices. This is especially true for women, where the spread of residual health scores over Social Network Index levels contracts as the assumed variance increases from 10 to 40 percent, and the relationship between health and social network scores loses statistical significance if the error variance is 20 percent or more. For men, the relationship remains significant at the .05 level up to 30 percent and remains less than .10 even at the maximum of 40 percent error; the spread of scores does not change appreciably from one error level to the next for men. These results suggest that the social network-subsequent health relationship among women must be treated with some reservations, depending on the validity of the health measure.

SOCIOECONOMIC STATUS, SOCIAL NETWORKS,
AND RESIDUAL HEALTH SCORES

As discussed in Chapter 4, there is ample evidence that social networks vary to some extent with socioeconomic status. Because socioeconomic status is also consistently predictive of health status, the former may be a confounding variable in the social network–health change relationship.

Interestingly enough, of the two socioeconomic status variables used in this analysis, only income is significantly associated with Social Network Index scores. Virtually no relationship exists between years of school completed and Social Network Index scores in 1965 for this group of respondents. Therefore, education would be unlikely to "explain away" the social network–health status association as might at least theoretically be anticipated in the case of income. The interrelationships of education, social networks, and subsequent health status should be examined, however, because there could be additive or interactive effects of the two risk variables.

The data in Table 6-10 show that despite the relationship between social ties and income, each still has an independent relationship to health. Persons with inadequate or marginal incomes fall below the expected follow-up health status score, but the size of the negative residual decreases steadily as social network scores increase. At the highest income level, on the other hand, all groups have a positive mean residual health score, indicating better health than predicted. Those who are also in the higher social network categories score more than twice as high on the follow-up health measure as those with lower social network scores. Among persons with "adequate" incomes, those with the lowest network scores have negative residual health scores, and those at the upper end of the Social Network Index have positive residual health scores in 1974. The adjusted health score for the "medium" network group at this income level is unexpectedly high. However, if the medium and medium-high categories are combined, the gradient for this group with adequate incomes smooths out. It may be that the distinction between the two middle categories is too fine a discrimination for reliable results in this three-variable analysis.

Looking at this part of Table 6-10 the other way around, one can see that the income effect persists at all levels of social connectedness; adjusted health scores improve steadily with rising income in each of the four social network score categories.

The two-way hierarchical analysis of variance shows that the effects of each of the two main risk variables are highly significant statistically and that there are not significant interaction effects. The fact that the range of health scores from the low income–low social network group (−1.76) to the high income–high network group (.49) is more than twice as great as the ranges associated with either risk variable alone, demonstrates that the effects of income and social network on future health are cumulative.

The additive effects of schooling and social networks on future health are equally clear. All those with less than 12 years of schooling, as well as all those with the lowest social network scores, have negative residual health scores. Their health is, on the average, worse than predicted on the basis of age, sex, and 1965 health status. In both cases, however, the negative effect of one risk variable was increasingly modified as scores on the other risk variable improved. The education effects are clearer within

Table 6-10. Mean residual physical health score by Social Network Index controlling for income and years of schooling

A. Family income, Social Network Index, and mean residual change scores

1965 Family income (adjusted for size of household)	Social Network Index, 1965									
	Low		Medium		Medium-high		High		Total	
	Mean	N	Mean	N	Mean	N	Mean	N	Mean	N
Inadequate or marginal	−1.76	109	−.38	283	−.35	149	−.16	162	−.53	703
Adequate	−.42	138	.09	571	−.11	536	.05	598	−.02	1843
Very adequate	.20	63	.17	336	.46	413	.49	416	.38	1228

	Sum of squares	DF	Mean square	F-Ratio	P
Main effects	533.50	5	106.70	7.500	.001
Family income level, 1965	381.43	2	190.72	13.405	.001
Social Network Index, 1965	152.07	3	50.69	3.563	.014
Interaction of family income level and social network	107.43	6	17.91	1.258	.274
Residual	53,523.29	3762	14.23		
Total	54,164.22	3773	14.36		

B. Years of schooling, Social Network Index, and mean residual health scores

Years of schooling completed in 1965	Social Network Index, 1965									
	Low		Medium		Medium-high		High		Total	
	Mean	N	Mean	N	Mean	N	Mean	N	Mean	N
0–11	−1.55	93	−.69	299	−.45	272	−.68	282	−.70	946
12	−.46	126	.05	417	.28	380	.35	416	.16	1339
13 or more	−.22	105	.24	532	.17	462	.55	497	.28	1596

	Sum of squares	DF	Mean square	F-Ratio	P
Main effects	809.69	5	161.94	11.340	.001
Years of schooling, 1965	626.68	2	313.34	21.942	.001
Social Network Index, 1965	183.01	3	61.00	4.272	.005
Interaction of years of schooling and social network	44.92	6	7.49	.524	.790
Residual	55,250.19	3869	14.28		
Total	56,104.81	3880	14.46		

each network category than they were within health practices categories; only in the medium-high group does one observe the reversal by which the health score actually declines with education beyond grade 12. This as well as the other minor irregularities in the middle network categories are smoothed out when the medium and medium-high scores are combined. In any case, it is clear that social network scores are associated with subsequent health at all educational levels, and number of years of schooling also predicts future health at all levels of social interaction. The main effects of both independent variables are seen to be highly significant, and no significant interaction effects are observed. Again, the range of future health scores obtained by classifying the sample on these two risk variables together is more than twice as great as that observed over categories of either education or networks alone, indicating that these two risk factors operate in an additive fashion in their influence on subsequent health.

Joint contribution of health practices and social networks to subsequent health status

This chapter has dealt with the health effects of two quite different aspects of life-style: health practices and social networks. The former consist essentially of behaviors directly related to the physical functioning of the organism, such as ingestion, exercise, and sleep. Social networks refer to a structure of social relationships within which an individual lives—a structure that may serve a wide range of physical, psychological, and social needs, either directly or indirectly.

The question that remains to be considered here is the relationship between health practices and social networks, and the nature of their combined impact on health. Do they represent independent risk factors that combine to have a greater impact on health than either would singly? Do they substitute for one another in some manner with one "explaining away" the impact of the other? Are there any kinds of special interaction effects of the two in relation to health?

THE RELATIONSHIP BETWEEN HEALTH PRACTICES AND SOCIAL NETWORKS

Do individuals with a large number of social connections have lower risk health practices than those who are relatively isolated? Do certain kinds of health-relevant practices such as excessive drinking, eating too much, or exercising too little affect the social connections that an individual maintains? Table 6-11 shows a positive association between Social Network Index scores and Health Practices Index scores in our sample.

Table 6-11. Distribution of 1965 Health Practices Index scores by 1965 Social Network Index scores

Health Practices Index	Social Network Index				
	Low (%)	Medium (%)	Medium-high (%)	High (%)	Total (%)
0–2	20.3	16.4	12.2	8.2	13.0
3	34.5	28.2	33.2	28.5	30.2
4	36.0	38.7	38.6	41.2	39.2
5	9.2	16.8	16.0	22.1	17.6
Total	100.0	100.1	100.0	100.0	100.0
N	325	1254	1116	1197	3892

Twenty percent of those in the lowest social network category report two or fewer good health habits compared to only 8 percent of those in the highest network group. Proportions in the middle range of health practices are fairly consistent over social network score groups, but only 9 percent of the least connected group report following all five good health practices whereas 22 percent of the most connected group so report. Chi-square tests indicate that the relationship between the two measures is significant at the .001 level.

THE JOINT CONTRIBUTION OF HEALTH PRACTICES
AND SOCIAL NETWORKS

Table 6-12 shows the follow-up residual health scores associated with various combinations of scores for our two measures of risk. These data reveal that the risks are additive. In general those with favorable scores on both measures seem maximally protected against negative health consequences, whereas those with unfavorable scores on both measures carry additional risk over that associated with either measure alone. The range of adjusted health scores in this cross-classification is greater than any seen in previous tables, including those that are cross-classified by socio-economic status variables. Hence the combination of these two factors—social networks and health practices—appears to be a powerful risk potential for future health. The analysis of variance shows that there are no significant interaction effects of the two independent variables.

Overall, the health score gradients in Table 6-12 follow the pattern observed in earlier cross-classifications; that is, within a given category on one risk factor, there is a generally steady gradient of residual health scores over the categories of the other risk factor, the health scores improving with higher life-style factor scores. At each successively higher level of a risk factor, this entire gradient shifts in a favorable direction. In Table 6-12 some exceptions to this may be seen. Within the group who report five low-risk health practices, there is no clear gradient by social network score.

There is some evidence that the influence of health practices on health is somewhat greater than that of social networks, as they are measured here. For instance, no matter what the level of social ties, the fact of practicing five low-risk health habits is enough to produce a positive residual health score, meaning that the 1974 health status score was better than predicted on the basis of 1965 health, age, and sex. The same is true for those who practice four of the five health habits at all but the very lowest social network level. However, even the largest system of social networks is not adequate to produce a positive residual health score in the presence of low health practices scores; groups scoring 3 or lower on the Health Practices Index all have negative residual health scores, although the impact of social networks can still be seen in the decreasing size of the negative scores with successively higher levels of social connectedness. The difference in impact of these two risk variables is also reflected in the

Table 6-12. Mean residual physical health score by Health Practices Index and Social Network Index

Social Network Index score, 1965	Index of Health Practices, 1965									
	0–2		3		4		5		Total	
	Mean	N	Mean	N	Mean	N	Mean	N	Mean	N
Low	−1.91	66	−.92	112	−.19	117	.80	30	−.70	325
Medium	−.62	206	−.43	353	.36	485	.18	210	−.06	1254
Medium-high	−.87	136	−.03	370	.27	431	.41	179	.06	1116
High	−.49	98	−.06	341	.22	493	.74	265	.20	1197
Total	−.83	506	−.24	1176	.25	1526	.48	684	.00	3829

Analysis of variance summary	Sum of squares	DF	Mean square	F-Ratio	P
Main effects	803.76	6	133.96	9.376	.001
Social Network Index, 1965	134.21	3	44.74	3.131	.025
Health Practices Index, 1965	593.27	3	197.76	13.841	.001
Interaction of social network and health practices	123.95	9	13.77	.964	.468
Residual	55,380.28	3876	14.29		
Total	56,307.99	3891	14.47		

analysis of variance summary, which shows a somewhat stronger significance ratio for health habits than for social networks.

The important finding in these data is that both health practices and social networks are strongly related to subsequent health, independent of each other and of socioeconomic status.

References

Belloc NB: Relationship of health practices and mortality. *Prev. Med.* **2**:67–81, 1973.

Belloc NB, Breslow L: Relationship of physical health status and health practices. *Prev. Med.* **1**:409–421, 1972.

Belloc NB, Breslow L, Hochstim JR: Measurement of physical health in a general population survey. *Am. J. Epidemiol.* **93**:328–336, 1971.

Bereiter C: Some presisting dilemmas in the measurement of change, in Harris C (ed): *Problems in Measuring Change*. Madison, University of Wisconsin Press, 1967, pp. 3–20.

Chafetz ME, et al: *Alcohol and Health*. U.S. Dept. of Health, Education and Welfare, Public Health Service, June 1974.

Graham S: Social factors in the relation to chronic illness, in Freeman HE, Levine S, Reeder LG, (eds): *Handbook of Medical Sociology*. Englewood Cliffs, N.J., Prentice-Hall, 1963, pp. 65–98.

Hochstim JR, Athanasopoulos DA, Larkins JH: Poverty area under the microscope. *Am. J. Public Health* **58**:1815–1827, 1968.

Hochstim JR, Renne S: Reliability of response in a sociomedical population study. *Public Opinion Q.* **35**:69–79, 1971.

Khosla T, Lowe CR: Obesity and smoking habits by social class. *J. Prev. Soc. Med.* **26**:249–256, 1972.

Meltzer JW, Hochstim JR: Reliability and validity of survey data on physical health. *Public Health Rep.* **85**:1075–1086, 1970.

National Center for Health Statistics: *Selected Health Characteristics by Occupation* Series 10, No. 21, Washington, D.C., 1965.

Palmore E: Health practices, illness, and longevity, in Palmore E, Jeffers F (eds): *Prediction of Life-Span*. Lexington, Mass., Heath Lexington Books, 1971, pp. 71–77.

Pesznecker BL, McNeil J: Relationship among health habits, social assets, psychological well-being, life change, and alterations in health status. *Nurs. Res.* **24**:442–447, 1975.

Pratt L: The relationship of socioeconomic status to health. *Am. J. Public Health* **62**:281–291, 1971.

Socioeconomic differentials in mortality. *Stat. Bull.* June 1972.

Syme LS, Berkman LF: Social class, susceptibility and sickness. *Am. J. Epidemiol.* **104**:1–8, 1976.

U.S. Dept. of Health, Education and Welfare: *Adult Use of Tobacco 1970*. Publ. No. HSM-73-8727, Washington, D.C., U.S. Government Printing Office, 1973.

Wiley JA, Camacho TC: Life-style and future health: Evidence from the Alameda County study. *Prev. Med.* **9**:1–21, 1980.

7. Summary and discussion

Introduction

In this monograph we have assembled data concerning health and ways of living from the Human Population Laboratory, Alameda County, California.

We have examined particularly the mortality among persons 30–69 years of age during the period 1965–1974 in relation to two aspects of living: (1) certain daily habits such as exercise, use of cigarettes, and alcohol; and (2) the nature and extent of social networks, that is, social connections in the form of marriage, close friends and relatives, church membership, and affiliation with nonchurch groups. In addition, one chapter covers the trend of physical health status, based on determinations in 1965 and again in 1974, in relation to the same two aspects of living.

Information about habits and social networks came from a questionnaire completed by a sample of the Alameda County adult population in 1965. The questionnaire also included queries concerning their physical, mental, and social well-being as well as their social and demographic characteristics. Follow-up of deaths among the population sample during the ensuing 9 years permitted analysis of how ways of living were associated with mortality.

An early report from the HPL had shown a strong association between physical health status in 1965 and certain habits termed *health practices*. Mortality checks through 1970 had revealed the association of these same health practices with deaths during the period 1965–1970. With further follow-up and the determination in 1974 of physical health status among survivors of the 1965 sample, it was possible to examine whether an association existed between health practices and social networks on the one hand, and the trend in health status as well as mortality between 1965 and 1974 on the other.

Thus we have considered two health "end points"—mortality and trend in physical health status—both over a 9-year period. And we have analyzed these in relation to two aspects of living: common personal health practices and social networks.

Conceptual framework

The significance of this work comes from the idea that health and disease arise mainly from circumstances of living. Within rather well-defined biologic limits, the health, disease, and mortality pattern of any community generally reflects the conditions of life in that community. Rural communities with poor sanitation located in areas heavily infested by parasites, mosquitoes, and other disease agents and vectors are afflicted with one pattern of health, disease, and mortality. Urban communities starting on the path of industrialization but affected by crowding, inadequate food, and poor sanitation have another pattern. Modern metropolitan communities with advanced industrialization and reasonably good sanitation, but low physical demand coupled with access to plenty of fatty foods, alcohol, and cigarettes, have still a third kind of health, disease, and mortality pattern.

Ways of living in the latter kind of community, just as in the others, underlie the typical health picture found there. Hence, ascertaining specific ways of living that are responsible for the health impairment and premature deaths that occur (or, on the contrary, ways of living that favor health and longevity) may lead to advances in health care. Knowledge that exposure to such disease agents as Anopheles mosquitoes and malaria, snails and schistosomes, drags down the health of a community, opened the path to improvement in such communities. Rudimentary industrialization with accompanying inadequate nutrition, exhaustion, and overcrowding have usually brought misery and premature death from tuberculosis and other diseases and injuries to many people. Knowledge of these relationships has led to social improvement and a healthier life. Correspondingly, knowledge of the precise features of living that harm health and preclude enjoyment of life's potential in the modern communities of the United States and similar countries should lead to further advances in health.

This thought stimulated development of the HPL in Alameda County, California, a community typical of the United States in the late twentieth century. The first aim was to measure health in the sense of the World Health Organization definition, "physical, mental and social well-being." The second was to examine ways of living in such a community that might contribute to or detract from the health of its people.

One set of ways of living to be studied consisted of seven common habits, such as excessive use of alcohol and cigarette smoking. Early investigations based on the Alameda County data confirmed and extended what was already known about the relationship of obesity, cigarette smoking, excessive use of alcohol, and other habits to health and mortality. A summary health practices score, with one point for each of seven favorable health practices, correlated highly both with physical health status in 1965 and with longevity based on mortality during the next 5 years. For example, a man at age 45 who was observing six or seven of the health practices had a life expectancy of about 11 years more than that of a 45-year-old man with a health practices score of 3 or less.

Another aspect of living—namely, the nature and extent of a person's social network—also attracted attention as a possibly significant factor in health and longevity. Earlier work by others had shown, for example, that being married was more favorable to health than being divorced, single, or widowed. Moving from one community to another, and thereby breaking social ties, appeared adverse to health. Belonging to a church seemed favorable. The original design of the HPL had provided for study of these factors. Thus it became possible to examine the relationship of social networks to physical health and mortality.

According to the HPL concept, health consisted of the three probably interrelated dimensions of well-being: physical, mental, and social. Each of these three could be regarded as a spectrum, so that an individual could be located at certain points on all three spectra and these points would represent that person's degree of health. Thus, for example, at age 25 a person would likely fall toward one (the healthy) end of the Physical Health Spectrum, and at age 85 toward the other. Death means reaching the latter end of the spectrum. If these concepts reflect reality, and if health practices and social networks influence both physical health and mortality, then health practices and social networks should also influence one's progress over time on the Physical Health Spectrum. Persons selected at any one time would, as a whole, be expected to move during the ensuing decade toward the less healthy end. Would that average movement toward poorer health and ultimate death, however, be measurably retarded by favorable health practices and strong social networks? Would it be accelerated by poor health practices and weak social networks? The

HPL provided an opportunity to examine the issue by making available a questionnaire measure of people's physical health status in 1965, their mortality through 1974, and another measure of health status for the same people who survived to 1974 and completed a second questionnaire.

The HPL approach to health—that is, its measurement, what influences it, and, implicitly, how it may be improved—departs from the prevailing scientific focus on understanding the biologic mechanisms of disease as the way to advance health. Discovering the precise mechanisms by which cells become cancerous might well open the path toward some means of countering the development of cancer. The same rationale applies generally to other diseases that plague modern humanity. History demonstrates, however, that interventions can be quite effectively planned without completely understanding the biological mechanisms involved. For example, it now appears that the sanitary campaigns, social reforms, and nutrition programs of the nineteenth and early twentieth century had at least as much to do with overcoming tuberculosis, cholera, pellagra, and other infectious and noninfectious diseases as did the discovery of the tubercle bacillus and other pathogenic microorganisms, important as these discoveries were. These interventions were frequently based on associations found between contaminated water or dietary factors and disease outcomes without the precise identification of the causal agents involved.

One task for the health scientists, then, is to examine—as people generally do, but more systematically and with scientific rigor—precisely what ways of living preclude or enhance the possibility of maximum health and longevity. Health and ways of living are natural phenomena and as such they are subject to scientific investigation. The crudeness of our definitions, concepts, and methods of measuring these phenomena only makes the task more challenging, not less important. Advancing knowledge in this direction will, it is hoped, help people who are seeking a healthful style of living in modern, urban, industrialized communities. Developing a knowledge base for guiding such action broadly would carry us beyond such significant but particular items as that cigarette smoking in the early 1980s accounts for more than 300,000 premature deaths in the United States each year, and that excessive consumption of alcohol adds greatly to that toll.

The usefulness of data from the HPL studies, as in any scientific investigation, depends on the methods of data collection. Because of the nature of the investigations intended, the laboratory staff devoted the first 5 years essentially to developing and testing such methods. That preparatory work enabled them to proceed with data collection that was economical, represented accurately the adult population of Alameda

County, showed reliability and validity so far as these could be ascertained, and provided information making it possible to follow up the sample. All these points had to be assured to the highest possible, and certainly to a satisfactory, degree before starting on the main study in 1965.

Summary of findings

Of the 2229 men aged 30–69 years constituting a 1965 sample of men that age in Alameda County, 9.5 percent died during the period 1965–1974. On the other hand, only 6.4 percent of the 2496 women 30–69 years of age in the sample died in that same time period. That mortality picture is consistent with statistics concerning death among all Alameda County men and women of the same age at the time.

Health practices

Analysis of the data revealed five common habits to be strongly, and each one independently, associated with mortality during the 9 years of follow-up. These habits, called high-risk health practices, were (1) smoking cigarettes, (2) consuming excessive quantities of alcohol, (3) being physically inactive, (4) being obese or underweight, and (5) sleeping fewer than 7 or more than 8 hours per night.

Two additional habits, skipping breakfast and snacking rather than eating regular meals, had been shown in an earlier analysis to be associated with mortality. That earlier analysis covered 5½ years' experience in the entire adult population sample, including those under 30 and over 69 years of age. The analysis reported here indicates that, for persons aged 30–69 years, not eating breakfast and snacking do not carry as heavy a mortality risk as the other five health practices.

To construct a simple Health Practices Index for purposes of further analysis, each of the five favorable health practices (i.e., not smoking cigarettes, drinking alcohol moderately if at all, being physically active, maintaining moderate weight, and sleeping 7–8 hours per night) was given one point. These points added to a score of 0–5 for each person. Thus people with a score of 0–2 can be considered as following high-risk health practices; 4–5, low-risk, and 3, intermediate.

Persons following the various individual high-risk health practices experienced death rates 25–115 percent higher than persons who followed the corresponding low-risk practices. Mortality, however, showed a strikingly higher gradient with the Health Practices Index that summarized all five health practices for each person. Thus the death rate among men 30–49 years of age with a health practices score of 0–2 was 840 percent (8.4 times) as high as that among men the same age with a health practices score of 4–5. For men aged 50–59 and 60–69 the relative risks were 2.4 and 1.7, respectively. As with practically all risk factor analyses among men, the association was stronger for younger men. Among women the corresponding relative risks in the three age groups (30–49, 50–59, and 60–69) were 2.9, 2.0, and 4.0, respectively.

These data confirm the strong relationship between number of health practices followed and mortality found in earlier analyses of the HPL data. Interpretation of that association, however, is by no means obvious. Persons who were seriously ill in 1965, and thus likely to die in the ensuing few years, may already have been unable to maintain normal weight, to exercise, or to sleep regularly 7–8 hours per night. A low health practices score hence might have reflected poor health and the likelihood of early death, rather than having preceded—and possibly been causally related to—mortality. Do "poor health practices" result in fatal illness or vice versa?

If profound and soon-to-be-fatal illness in 1965 had been largely responsible for the low health practices scores in the sample, then the deaths associated with those low scores should have occurred mainly among persons who were already disabled in 1965, persons so sick as to be unable to exercise, or maintain normal weight, and whose sleep was disturbed, and among those who died in the first years of the follow-up period.

In fact, the data do not support that hypothesis. Among men, an even steeper mortality gradient prevailed among those with no health problems and those with only symptoms than among persons who reported some chronic conditions and disability of varying degrees. Also, during the period 1965–1974, less than one-seventh of the male deaths occurred among the 5 percent who had any disability and a Health Practices Index of 0–3 in 1965. Finally, only a small minority of the deaths in that group occurred during the first 1½ years of the follow-up, when seriously ill people would have been likely to die. Though there was a slight concentration during the early years, the deaths were distributed fairly evenly over all 9 years.

Thus the striking association between health practices and mortality cannot be explained by preexisting disease resulting in the "poor health practices."

Analysis of the data reveals, moreover, that the health practices score predicts mortality independently of socioeconomic status, race, and seven psychological factors examined. Finally, the Health Practices Index is related not only to total mortality, but strongly also to death rates from each of four major categories of disease: coronary heart disease, cerebrovascular and other circulatory disease, cancer, and all other diseases.

Social networks

Several items in the questionnaire were used as a measure of the nature and extent of social connections in the form of marriage, contacts with close friends and relatives, church membership, and affiliation with non church groups. The HPL mortality rates showed a gradient with each of the four components of the social network. For example, the age-adjusted mortality among unmarried men aged 30–69 was 14.7, compared with 8.4 among married men. The corresponding rates among women were 7.6 and 5.8. Mortality among the men with few close friends and relatives was 12.5, but only 7.4 among men with many close friends and relatives; corresponding rates among women were 11.2 and 4.6.

To investigate their cumulative relationship to mortality, the four types of social connections were used to construct a Social Network Index. The latter divided the study population into four groups: I (fewest connections), II, III, and IV (most connections).

This Social Network Index showed a gradient with mortality: group I had the highest death rate and group IV the lowest. The mortality gradient with Social Network Index was just about as striking as with the Health Practices Index. Men constituting the most isolated group had an age-adjusted mortality rate 2.3 times higher than men with the strongest social connections; among women the difference was 2.8 times.

As with the Health Practices Index, the association of the Social Network Index with mortality persisted through all degrees of the Physical Health Spectrum and concentrated only to a minor extent in the early years of follow-up. Thus it could not be explained on the basis of pre-existing disease. Likewise, the Social Network Index revealed a mortality gradient with all of the major groups of disease: coronary heart disease, cerebrovascular and other circulatory disease, cancer, and all other diseases. Quite uniformly, for both sexes, those with a stronger social network had lower death rates than those with weaker ties.

Because a person's social network is obviously related to that individual's position in the social structure, we examined social class, race, level of urbanization, geographic mobility, and occupational mobility as possibly confounding variables. All of these had been shown by other investigators to be associated both with social networks and with health. Analysis was therefore directed toward (1) ascertaining the relationship between each of the sociostructural elements (social class and others) and social networks; and (2) assessing whether the Social Network Index predicted mortality independently of the other social factors.

Many studies show an association between socioeconomic status and health. Data from the HPL confirm that association. The latter also reveal, however, that throughout the socioeconomic spectrum men and women with few social contacts had higher mortality rates than those with many connections. This finding supports the conclusion that the Social Network Index predicts mortality independently of socioeconomic status. Analysis also indicated that the relationship between social isolation and mortality risk could not be attributed to race, geographic mobility, occupational mobility, or level of urbanization so far as these could be measured from the questionnaires. The social network gradient in mortality likewise persisted through the varying levels of preventive health care.

It is often suggested that psychological states may either mediate the relationship between social networks and mortality or affect people's network directly. According to the first hypothesis, people without social ties become lonely, depressed, or otherwise psychologically disturbed and some such state induces disease. According to the second hypothesis, people who are psychologically disturbed find it difficult to maintain social ties.

In order to explore these issues, the psychological characteristics ascertained in the 1965 survey were analyzed. Seven of these factors, including personal uncertainty, anomy, and life satisfaction, were selected. Of them, the one termed life satisfaction proved to be most significant for predicting mortality, the relative risk being almost 2 for men and 3 for women. Nevertheless, the Social Network Index was associated with mortality independently of life satisfaction, as well as the other six psychological factors examined.

Thus the findings indicate that the extent to which people maintain social connections is strongly associated with risk of mortality. The relationship holds independently of age, physical health status at baseline, position in social structure including socioeconomic status, level of preventive health care, and the seven psychological factors that were examined.

The association between health practices, social networks, and mortality is clear. And it appears to be independent of possibly confounding factors such as age, sex, race, physical health status at baseline, preventive health care, and socioeconomic status, when these factors are considered one at a time. The possibility that, cumulatively, these factors might account for the association was also examined, using multiple logistic analysis. The latter method confirmed the independence of the associations between mortality and the health practices and social networks. When considering all potential confounders (including both social networks and health practices) simultaneously in the logistic analysis, the approximate relative mortality risk for those with many high-risk health practices was 2.4 for men and 2.2 for women. For those with least social contacts, the risks were 2.2 and 2.4 for men and women, respectively.

Both sets of factors were also found to be associated in the expected direction, with changes in health status occurring between 1965 and 1974. As anticipated, physical health status for the sample population as a whole declined over the 9-year period, consistent with aging of the population. The decline was significantly greater, however, among those who were following high-risk health practices, had weak social networks in 1965, or both; correspondingly, the decline was significantly less among persons with low-risk health practices and strong social networks. These associations are independent not only of each other but also of socioeconomic status.

In summary, the data substantiate early findings of the HPL that health is associated with certain common habits called health practices, and with social networks. The associations are strong and prevail not only with regard to health status as originally determined in the 1965 survey, but also through 9 years of mortality experience, and through decline of physical health status over the same time period. Persons with high-risk health practices and weak social networks die off more rapidly and their physical health deteriorates faster. The associations of these two sets of ways of living persist in all four major categories of causes of death, as well as in mortality as a whole. They are independent of—that is, cannot be "explained by"—age, sex, socioeconomic status, baseline physical health, and other potentially confounding factors examined.

Discussion

The findings summarized above and presented in detail in the earlier chapters confirm the relationship between health and what people do in their daily lives. Also they raised many issues that cannot be directly answered by further analyses of these data. Some of these questions have to do with social networks: How are social networks related to health status? What is it about social isolation that carries health consequences? What are the biologic mechanisms that lead from social disconnection to disease and death? Other similar questions concern the relationships between health habits and morbidity and mortality, though we are closer to understanding how certain physical aspects of living, such as exposure to cigarette smoke, affect health.

What can be clearly perceived is the historical relationship between ways of living and the patterns of health, disease, and mortality. During the early stages of industrialization, the conditions of life among the increasing numbers of people who were being drawn into factory work obviously affected health and mortality. Major determinants were the physical conditions of life such as grossly poor sanitation, polluted water, crowding, and impaired access to food. Later stages of industrialization have brought relative affluence to masses of people. This relative affluence has made rich food, cigarettes, and alcohol widely available and attractive; it has also reduced the physical demands of life. In addition, advanced industrial civilization, especially in the United States, has profoundly changed family patterns and other social relationships.

It now appears that these alterations in ways of living may be fundamentally responsible for the contrasting patterns of disease in the two periods. In the latter part of the nineteenth and early twentieth centuries, tuberculosis and other respiratory infections, as well as typhoid and other intestinal infections, dominated the scene. In the latter part of the twentieth century, their place has been taken by coronary and other cardiovascular diseases, lung cancer, and other forms of noninfectious respiratory disease. About midway through the twentieth century when this changed pattern was recognized, it seemed to many that cancer and cardiovascular disease were occurring as a "natural" concomitant of aging. Now it is becoming evident that ways of living still determine the disease picture, that premature deaths in our type of society generally reflect, among other things, cigarette smoking, excessive consumption of alcohol, and other common habits termed health practices in this volume; and by what are here termed weak social networks. A perspective in which chronic diseases are not viewed as an inevitable part of the aging process invites efforts to extend both the life span and years of life free from disability. Such a view now seems justifiable; in fact, evidence is mounting that many of the physiological changes we commonly think of as part of the "natural aging process" are to a large degree environmentally determined.

The etiologic issue

The etiologic question is whether the associations disclosed by this research are causal, and what can be done to examine that inference. Epidemiologic data of the sort presented do not themselves "establish" or "prove" causality. The latter is a matter of judgment. Understanding and specifying the biologic mechanisms involved, though often highly useful, are not essential to making judgments about causality, except in a very narrow sense. That view is especially pertinent to situations in which multiple etiologies exist. Thus one can now say that cigarette smoking causes lung cancer and should be avoided in order to prevent that disease, even though we only vaguely comprehend the biologic mechanisms of the etiology and realize that other (multiple) agents can also cause the disease.

Some points supporting a judgment of causality have been presented with the data. One involves the strength of the associations; their over-whelming statistical significance, that is, the probability of their being true associations rather than due to chance; and their independence from several possibly confounding factors such as age, sex, and socioeconomic status.

Another is the temporal sequence: The high-risk health practices and weak social network configurations appear to precede serious illness. Thus the associations apparently cannot be explained on the basis that those who died were already very sick and thus could not exercise, sleep regularly, or maintain social relationships.

The associations found are substantially consistent with a large body of other data. Many individual components of the health practices and social network analyzed in the Alameda County studies, such as cigarette smoking and being separated or divorced, are well known to be associated with premature mortality. Using alcohol to excess damages the liver and other organs and often leads to accidents. Segments of the population that generally follow low-risk health practices and maintain strong social networks, such as Mormons and Seventh Day Adventists, have much lower mortality than the population as a whole.

Obviously, it would be useful in interpreting the Alameda County data to have other sets of essentially comparable information in order to ascertain whether the results are consistent. That would add to the foundation for inferences. Additionally, it would be helpful to have more data on the incidence and case fatality of specific diseases so that the "generality hypothesis" could be tested more accurately. Incidence data would also provide important clues as to where along the spectrum of disease health practices and social networks have their greatest impacts.

The intervention issue

Whether or not to take action designed to improve health practices and strengthen social networks as a means of enhancing health should, of course, be determined by careful assessment and interpretation. For certain of the five individual health practices, judgment has already been made and action initiated.

One fundamental characteristic of the modern ways of living examined here for their relationship to health appears on the surface to differentiate them from the key health-related factors of early industrial civilization.

The latter required broad social action as the main strategy: to achieve general sanitation and healthful water, to improve housing and food supplies. Dealing with habits and social relationships—that is, behavior— as a means of advancing health has commonly been thought to require individual action. In effect, each person decides each day, usually habitually, of course, how much exercise and sleep to obtain, whether to continue living with a spouse or to see the in-laws. Perhaps nowhere is this view better articulated than in a paper by Knowles (1977) entitled *The responsibility of the individual.*

The individual has the power—indeed the moral responsibility—to maintain his own health by the observance of simple prudent rules of behavior relating to sleep, exercise, diet and weight, alcohol and smoking. In addition he should avoid where possible the long-term use of drugs. He should be aware of the dangers of stress and the need for precautionary measures during periods of sudden change, such as bereavement, divorce, or new employment. He should submit to selective medical examination and screening procedures. (p. 80)

Obviously, individuals should be encouraged to make decisions in these matters that are favorable to their health. Yet there are serious limitations to approaching behavioral change from such an individualistic perspective. Paramount is the fact that individuals begin and maintain behaviors within a certain social, psychological, and cultural context. These behaviors do not occur randomly throughout a population, nor do they occur in a vacuum. Powerful social influences bear on them. The evidence of these influences is clearest with regard to smoking.

Early research efforts focused on why particular individuals started or were unable to stop smoking, on "oral needs," neuroticism, and insecurity among smokers. The powerful social and environmental pressures influencing smoking behavior were relatively neglected. As time went on, however, it became apparent that whether a person smokes depends on whether that person's friends, parents, and siblings smoke; on how the media projects smokers; and on a person's information concerning the health effects of smoking (Syme and Alcalay, 1982). The fact that most smokers understand that cigarettes are harmful to health—for instance, 92 percent of teenagers agree that "cigarette smoking can harm the health of teenagers" (Fishbein, 1977)—underscores the importance of subtle forces that make smoking an attractive behavior.

Whereas smoking is a habit that initially has strong extrinsic or social influences, in time it develops its own intrinsic motivations and rewards. Thus the habit both reflects certain social and cultural norms and expectations, and provides a certain pleasure. Dependence ensues. Smoking may also be seen as a kind of coping behavior in which people rely on cigarettes to provide relief from stressful situations. Job stresses, divorce, family conflicts, loneliness, and other anxious and tense situations have all been reported by smokers to increase cigarette consumption. Smoking may be a way to "control" negative feelings and disturbances (Benfari et al., 1982). The Alameda County data showed that people who were lacking many social and community contacts were more likely to be smokers.

Even in this brief review we see that smoking is a complex behavior motivated by forces that are social, cultural, and psychological. Other behaviors such as alcohol consumption, eating patterns, and physical exercise may be formed and maintained by such forces as well. Sleep patterns or disturbances have traditionally been viewed as reflecting environmental and psychological stresses. Intervention strategies that ignore the causes of behaviors and focus on the individual's ability to control behavior in the face of considerable environmental obstacles are likely to fail. On the other hand, environmental interventions that are preventive and alter the social forces that motivate people to smoke, drink heavily, and maintain other high-risk behaviors seem more promising.

The actions required to induce health-promoting behavior cannot be regarded as matters of purely individual responsibility. On ethical grounds, therefore, social action to influence health-related behavioral decisions is necessary. On sheer economic grounds, when dealing with a problem of such magnitude, social interventions will be more practical and efficient than individualized programs.

Furthermore, the behavior of one person can affect the health of other members of society. The hazard of being injured by a drunken driver is a risk to all of us, and we all share the cost of medical care and other social debits for that same alcohol-intoxicated person.

The health of a society is built not only upon sound medicine and good hospitals and physicians, but upon the preventive actions taken to insure the health and well-being of all its members. Health risks confronting us today require that we think more creatively and develop new preventive strategies to deal with the social and behavioral causes of disease.

References

Benfari R, Ockene JK, McIntyre KM: Control of cigarette smoking from a psychological perspective. *Ann. Rev. Public Health* 3:101–128, 1982.

Fishbein M: Consumer beliefs and behavior with respect to cigarette smoking: a critical analysis of the public literature. In *Federal Trade Commission Report to Congress: Pursuant to the Public Health Cigarette Smoking Act.* Washington, D.C., Federal Trade Commission, 1977.

Knowles, JH: The responsibility of the individual. *Daedalus*, Winter 1977, pp. 57–80.

Syme SL, Alcalay R: Control of cigarette smoking from a social perspective. *Ann. Rev. Public Health* 3:179–199, 1982.

Appendix

The Human Population Laboratory, in its attempt to measure "mental well-being" in the Alameda County residents, asked a variety of psychological questions on the 1965 survey. These items were contained in five major indices: (1) a 19-item index of "ego resiliency"; (2) a 20-item index of "neurotic traits"; (3) a nine-item index of "anomy"; (4) an index of eight items measuring positive and negative feelings; and (5) an index comprised of four items describing being bothered or dissatisfied with certain social roles. Since many of these indices are of unknown validity and/or were created specifically for the HPL survey, a factor analysis of all items from the psychological indices were conducted. This analysis verified the unidimensionality of psychological variables used in this examination. A brief history of the origins of the HPL indices follows.

The first index, measuring "ego resiliency," was advanced by Block (1965) at one stage of his work which eventually culminated in his volume on response sets. Block defined resiliency as "resourcefulness, adaptability, and engagement in the world"; he used the term ego to imply that "an enduring structural aspect of the individual is involved." The term ego resiliency was therefore intended to "denote the individual's characteristic capability when under the strain set by new environmental demands."

The neurotic traits index has five subscales of four items each, measuring isolation, dissatisfaction, immobilization, perfectionism, and impulsiveness. This index has been reported to be related to ego strength.

The index of anomy was developed by McCloskey and Schaar (1965) and has been extensively described and validated. Its purpose is to measure "a sense of normlessness" relating to a wide variety of cognitive and personality factors as well as to the more traditional social factors generally associated with anomy. In particular, the scale is correlated with hostility, anxiety, inflexibility, and defensiveness.

Perhaps the best known of the psychological variables is an eight-item index of positive and negative feelings. This scale was developed by Bradburn and Caplovitz (1965) to measure psychological well-being. The HPL index, however, is not identical to the Bradburn-Caplovitz index, since it omits one item, i.e., "feeling proud because someone complimented you on something you had done," and also has a longer time-span referent than the original. Thus, the HPL index is not precisely validated by previous work done with the Bradburn-Caplovitz scale. The eight-item HPL index, however, has been reported by P. Berkman (1971) to measure the same psychological dimension as that identified by the psychiatric ratings done in the Midtown Manhattan Study (1971).

Finally, the last index attempts to measure whether or not an individual's expectations in four major life roles have been fulfilled and, if not, whether the individual is bothered by the lack of fulfillment. The four roles are: provider, worker, marital partner, and parent. Though these items appear to have a great deal of face validity, they were items created for the HPL survey and have undergone no rigorous tests of validity.

Because many of the psychological indices in the Human Population Laboratory survey were of unknown validity, and since several previous analyses on some of these indices had shown them not to be unidimensional, it was decided to conduct a factor analysis of the entire set of psychological items. This method was used to construct indices based on observed relationships in the data which could then be used in the prediction of mortality. Rather than reflecting theoretical positions as the original indices did, these new variables are reflections of empirical correlations found among individual items (Cattell, 1965). These clusters of items are formed into factors which then can be transformed into indices. If the original indices were accurate measures of psychological dimensions which are unidimensional, these dimensions should remain intact through the factor analysis and emerge as a new factor.

Factor analysis subsumes a variety of procedures so that decisions must be made during the analysis process about which procedures will most appropriately fit the data and the needs of the investigator. The procedures will be discussed as well as the rationale for choosing them. The computer program used in all these analyses is the Statistical Package for the Social Sciences (SPSS) (Nie et al., 1975).

The first step in the analysis after the preparation of the correlation matrix of all psychological items was the extraction of initial factors. This was done by a classical factor analysis instead of a principal component analysis. This seemed to be a more realistic method, since it was based on the assumption that the observed correlations were mainly the results of some underlying regularity in the data.

After the initial factors were selected, they were rotated in one of several ways into terminal factors so that simpler and theoretically more meaningful factor patterns emerged. In this analysis, an oblique rotation was used instead of an orthogonal one. This method was chosen because the underlying dimensions were not assumed to be unrelated to one other, an assumption made with orthogonal rotation. This method more accurately shows how variables cluster together, since the rotating axes can come closer to each respective cluster of variables. Also, the oblique solution provides information about the actual amount of correlation among factors. Table A-1 shows the correlations among the seven factors formed from the psychological items.

A maximum number of seven factors was specified to result from the factor analysis. The percent of variance and cumulative percent of variance accounted for by each of the seven factors is shown in Table A-2. As seen in the table, the first factor accounts for over half the variance among items and the last two factors account for only a small proportion, under 5%, of the total variance.

The final step in the analysis was the construction of indices from the seven factors. For each factor, a list of items was developed based on their degree of correlation with the factor. All items whose correlations were under .20 were immediately dropped from the developing index. The remaining cut-off points were based on theoretical considerations in which it appeared that the meaning of the factor would be significantly changed by the inclusion of items below a certain correlation. Once the

Table A-1. Correlations among seven psychological factors

Factor	1	2	3	4	5	6	7
1	1.00						
2	.26	1.00					
3	−.22	−.17	1.00				
4	.31	.26	.15	1.00			
5	.39	.20	.10	.28	1.00		
6	.43	.08	−.19	.16	.28	1.00	
7	.18	.12	.23	.19	.27	.15	1.00

Table A-2. Percent of variance accounted for by factors

Factor	Percent of variance	Cumulative percentage
1	52.7	52.7
2	13.9	66.6
3	8.9	75.5
4	8.6	84.1
5	6.8	91.0
6	4.8	95.8
7	4.2	100.0

cut-off point was determined, however, in no cases were items below that degree of correlation included in the index or items above that point excluded.

The new factors, each comprised of ten or fewer items, were then scored so that each item was weighted equally and scores for each factor were simply the cumulative responses to the ten items. The cumulative scores were divided approximately into thirds so that the bottom third represented low scores on the index, middle scores were labeled medium, and the top third scored high on the index. Finally, each individual's score was calculated according to the percentage of items answered. For example, an individual who had a total of two points from answering only four of six items on a particular index received the same score as someone who scored three points but answered all six questions, i.e., $2/4 = 3/6$. Individuals who did not respond to half or more of the items in an index were called nonrespondents and were dropped from the analyses. This resulted in the loss of very few individuals, generally less than 1% of the sample.

Factor 1, personal uncertainty

The first factor, which accounts for over half the variance in the factor analysis, is comprised of seven questions, six of which are from the neurotic traits index. The final item is from the McCloskey and Schaar anomy scale. These items are all scored true or false with two points being given for a true response and one point for a false response. The items are as follows:

1. "I am easily sidetracked from things I start to do."
2. "I have a hard time making up my mind about things I should do."
3. "I keep putting things off, and I don't get as much done as others do."

4. "Much of the time I'm not sure what I really want."
5. "I have periods of days, weeks, or months when I can't get going."
6. "I often do things on the spur of the moment without stopping to think."
7. "It seems to me that other people find it easier to decide what is right than I do."

Factor 2, anomy, normlessness

The second factor is comprised entirely of anomy items. It includes seven of the original nine questions, omitting two which appear to be more personally or internally oriented. The remaining items seem to reflect a more worldly or external normlessness. It has also been suggested that these items reflect a traditionalist attitude or feeling that "the world was better off in the good old days." This suggestion is given some support by the observation that this factor, more than any other, is strongly associated with age. The seven items, which were scored true and false identically to Factor 1, were:

1. "With everything in such a state of disorder, it's hard for a person to know where he stands from one day to the next."
2. "People were better off in the old days when everyone knew just how he was expected to act."
3. "What is lacking in the world today is the old kind of friendship that lasted for a lifetime."
4. "The trouble with the world today is that most people really don't believe in anything."
5. "I often feel that many things our parents stood for are just going to ruin before our very eyes."
6. "With everything so uncertain these days, it almost seems as though anything could happen."
7. "Everything changes so quickly these days that I often have trouble deciding which are the right rules to follow."

Factor 3, life satisfaction

Items from five different indices comprise Factor 3, which has been termed a measure of life satisfaction. No other factor in analysis drew from so many different indices. It is made up of nine items, including all the positive feeling items from the Bradburn-Caplovitz index and three questions concerning satisfaction in major life roles:

1. "How often do you feel on top of the world?"
2. "All in all, how happy are you these days?"

3. "How often do you feel particularly excited or interested in something?"
4. "How often do you feel pleased about having accomplished something?"
5. "Has your marriage turned out to be better or worse than you expected?"
6. "On the whole life gives me a lot of pleasure."
7. "I feel as good now as I ever have."
8. "Have your children turned out to be better or worse than expected?"
9. "Considering everything, how satisfied are you with your present job?"

All of these items were scored on a scale of 1 to 3. Items 1, 3, and 4 were scored: (1) never, (2) sometimes, (3) often. Items 5 and 8 were scored: (1) worse, (2) about the same, (3) better. Item 9 was scored: (1) not satisfied, (2) somewhat satisfied, and (3) very satisfied. Items 6 and 7 were scored: (1) false, (2) true. The second item on happiness was scored: (1) not so happy, (2) pretty happy, (3) very happy. Low scores on this index were a reflection of people who reported little satisfaction; high scorers, conversely, were those who reported much life satisfaction.

Factor 4, social insecurity

Factor 4 appears to be comprised of items representing social threat or insecurity. Most of the ten items in this index derive from the ego-resiliency index. The responses to all these items are either true or false with two points given to a true response and one point given to a false one. This is true with the exception of item 7, in which one point is given for a true response and two for a false response. High scorers are therefore people who are less secure in the ways they interact with others; low scorers are more secure. In order of their degree of correlation, the ten items are:

1. "It's hard for me to start a conversation with strangers."
2. "I feel nervous if I have to meet a lot of people."
3. "I usually don't talk much unless I am with people I know very well."
4. "It is hard for me to act natural when I'm with new people."
5. "Clever, sarcastic people make me feel very uncomfortable."
6. "I often feel awkward and out of place."
7. "I think I am usually a leader in my group."
8. "I get very tense and anxious when I think other people are disapproving of me."
9. "Criticisms or scolding makes me very uncomfortable."
10. "Often when I'm with a group of people I feel left out even if they are friends of mine."

Factor 5, *perfectionism*

Three items form Factor 5. They were all on the neurotic traits index originally, and all come from the same subscale which the Human Population Laboratory has called a measure of perfectionism. The response to the items are true or false, with two points given to "true" responses and one to "false." People who scored high on the index, therefore, were more "perfectionistic" than those who scored low. The items were:

1. "Even when other people praise my work, I am still dissatisfied."
2. "I'm never quite satisfied with what I do."
3. "Almost every time I finish doing something, I feel I could have done it better."

Factor 6, *negative feelings*

Factor 6 is comprised of six items, five of which are negative feelings statements from the Bradburn-Caplovitz index. The final item is taken from the ego resiliency index. The six items are:

1. "How often do you feel depressed or very unhappy?"
2. "How often do you feel very lonely or remote from other people?"
3. "How often do you feel vaguely uneasy about something without knowing why?"
4. "How often do you feel bored?"
5. "How often do you feel so restless you couldn't sit long in a chair?"
6. "I get pretty discouraged sometimes."

The first five items were scored from 1 to 3 with a score of 1 equaling a response of "never," 2 being "sometimes," and 3 meaning "often." The sixth item was scored true/false, with a score of 3 being given to a "true" response and a score of 1 given to a "false" response. Thus, high scorers on this index reported the most negative feelings and low scorers the least.

Factor 7, *isolation-depression*

The final cluster of items seems to form a set of responses representing isolation or depression. Five of the six items are drawn from the neurotic traits index; the other item (5) comes from the ego resilency index:

1. "I tend to keep people at a distance."
2. "It's hard for me to feel close to others."
3. "I find it easy to drop or break with a friend."
4. "I don't enjoy many of the things other people seem to like."

5. "It often seems that my life has no meaning."
6. "Much of the time, I'm not sure what I really want."

These items were all scored true/false with one point given for a "false" response and two for a "true" response. People who scored high on this scale were therefore most isolated and people who scored low were least isolated or depressed.

Table A-3. Age-adjusted mortality rates from all causes (per 100): Social Network Index and Factor 1, personal uncertainty, men and women ages 30–69, 1965–1974

Social Network Index[a]	Level of personal uncertainty							
	Low	(N)	Medium	(N)	High	(N)	Total	(N)
Men								
I	6.9	(49)	17.7	(49)	20.5	(57)	15.1	(155)
II	11.0	(217)	11.2	(217)	14.4	(164)	12.0	(598)
III	9.6	(271)	9.6	(266)	9.8	(160)	8.5	(697)
IV	5.3	(338)	7.5	(292)	10.2	(131)	6.9	(761)
Total	7.1	(875)	9.8	(824)	12.8	(512)	9.4	(2211)
Women								
I	12.1	(77)	13.7	(89)	10.2	(104)	11.8	(270)
II	5.6	(231)	4.6	(298)	11.8	(326)	7.3	(855)
III	3.2	(171)	4.9	(232)	6.8	(197)	5.0	(600)
IV	5.0	(258)	2.7	(308)	6.0	(189)	4.3	(755)
Total	5.6	(737)	4.9	(927)	9..	(816)	6.4	(2480)

[a]Index ranges from I (least connections) to IV (most connections).

Table A-4. Age-adjusted mortality rates from all causes (per 100): Social Network Index and Factor 2, anomy, men and women ages 30–69, 1965–1974

Social Network Index[a]	Level of anomy							
	High	(N)	Medium	(N)	Low	(N)	Total	(N)
Men								
I	16.4	(54)	13.0	(59)	15.2	(40)	14.7	(153)
II	12.7	(189)	12.4	(252)	11.0	(155)	12.1	(596)
III	9.2	(189)	9.5	(264)	5.9	(244)	8.4	(697)
IV	6.2	(219)	7.6	(294)	6.3	(246)	6.8	(759)
Total (N)	9.8	(651)	9.7	(869)	10.6	(685)	9.3	(2205)
Women								
I	12.6	(120)	10.1	(85)	10.2	(66)	11.2	(271)
II	7.1	(301)	7.1	(316)	7.3	(240)	7.1	(857)
III	4.4	(171)	6.0	(229)	3.8	(198)	4.9	(598)
IV	4.6	(220)	5.2	(284)	2.6	(250)	4.3	(754)
Total (N)	5.2	(812)	6.8	(914)	5.2	(754)	6.3	(2480)

[a]Index ranges from I (least connections) to IV (most connections)

Table A-5. Age adjusted mortality rates from all causes (per 100): Social Network Index and Factor 4, social insecurity, men and women ages 30–69, 1965–1974

Social Network Index[a]	Level of social insecurity							
	High	(N)	Medium	(N)	Low	(N)	Total	(N)
Men								
I	18.6	(58)	12.1	(53)	12.3	(43)	14.7	(154)
II	10.5	(195)	14.7	(224)	9.9	(179)	11.9	(598)
III	6.9	(182)	9.8	(275)	7.8	(242)	8.5	(699)
IV	8.2	(173)	4.2	(287)	5.3	(303)	6.8	(763)
Total (N)	9.9	(608)	10.4	(839)	8.8	(767)	9.3	(2214)
Women								
I	10.5	(128)	11.5	(99)	17.2	(44)	11.7	(271)
II	7.8	(376)	7.0	(270)	6.8	(211)	7.3	(857)
III	5.0	(220)	4.5	(231)	5.4	(149)	5.0	(600)
IV	3.0	(198)	3.7	(291)	5.9	(267)	4.4	(756)
Total (N)	6.7	(922)	5.9	(891)	6.8	(671)	6.4	(2484)

[a]Index ranges from I (least connections) to IV (most connections).

Table A-6. Age-adjusted mortality rates from all causes (per 100): Social Network Index and Factor 5, perfectionism, men and women ages 30–69, 1965–1974

Social Network Index[a]	Level of perfectionism							
	High	(N)	Medium	(N)	Low	(N)	Total	(N)
Men								
I	19.4	(52)	10.4	(46)	14.6	(56)	14.7	(154)
II	10.8	(210)	11.2	(127)	13.6	(259)	11.9	(596)
III	9.1	(214)	8.6	(145)	8.2	(337)	8.5	(696)
IV	7.8	(220)	6.4	(182)	6.2	(359)	6.7	(761)
Total (N)	10.0	(696)	8.6	(500)	9.2	(1011)	9.3	(2207)
Women								
I	9.8	(86)	14.0	(51)	12.2	(134)	11.7	(271)
II	7.5	(273)	9.0	(170)	6.3	(412)	7.1	(855)
III	5.3	(149)	3.0	(112)	5.3	(338)	4.9	(599)
IV	4.9	(173)	4.7	(125)	3.8	(456)	4.3	(754)
Total	6.5	(681)	7.0	(458)	6.1	(1340)	6.4	(2479)

[a]Index ranges from I (least connections) to IV (most connections).

Table A-7. Age-adjusted mortality rates from all causes (per 100): Social Network Index and Factor 6, negative feelings, men and women ages 30–69, 1965–1974

Social Network Index[a]	Level of negative feelings							
	Low	(N)	Medium	(N)	High	(N)	Total	(N)
Men								
I	16.0	(42)	15.0	(50)	14.1	(62)	14.9	(154)
II	11.2	(177)	11.8	(204)	13.9	(215)	12.2	(596)
III	7.6	(248)	9.2	(247)	9.0	(206)	8.5	(701)
IV	4.7	(319)	9.0	(254)	6.7	(189)	6.9	(762)
Total (N)	7.6	(786)	10.2	(755)	11.3	(672)	9.4	(2213)
Women								
I	9.8	(63)	12.6	(81)	12.8	(129)	11.9	(273)
II	6.8	(185)	6.9	(295)	7.7	(376)	7.3	(856)
III	2.9	(148)	5.0	(225)	6.6	(227)	4.9	(600)
IV	3.9	(278)	4.3	(274)	5.1	(200)	4.3	(752)
Total (N)	5.1	(674)	6.4	(875)	7.9	(932)	6.4	(2481)

[a]Index ranges from I (least connections) to IV (most connections).

Index of marital adjustment

The marital adjustment index was developed based on the responses to nine questions:

1. Many women (men) feel that they are not as good wives (husbands) as they would like to be. How often have you felt this way?

   1. never 2. rarely 3. sometimes 4. often

2. Does your husband (wife) give you as much understanding as you need?

   1. no, not really 2. yes, but not completely, 3. yes, completely

3. Does your husband (wife) show you as much affection as you would like?

   1. more than I like 2. as much as I like 3. less than I like

4. Even happily married couples sometimes have problems getting along with each other. How often does this happen to you?

   1. often 2. sometimes 3. a few times 4. never

5. When you and your husband (wife) disagree, who usually gives in?

   1. I do 2. he does 3. other (what)

6. Do you ever regret your marriage?

   1. often 2. sometimes 3. a few times 4. never

7. Have you seriously considered separation or divorce recently?

   1. yes 2. no

8. All in all, how happy has your marriage been for you?

    1. very unhappy   2. unhappy   3. somewhat unhappy   4. somewhat happy
                  5. happy   6. very happy

9. Has your marriage turned out to be better or worse than you expected?

    1. better   2. about the same   3. worse

References

1. Berkman PL: Life stress and psychological well-being: A replication of Langner's analysis in the Midtown Manhattan Study. *J. Health Soc. Behav.* **12**:35–45, 1971.
2. Block J: *The Challenge of Response Sets.* New York, Appleton, 1965
3. Bradburn NM, Caplovitz D: *Reports on Happiness: A Pilot Study of Behavior Related to Mental Health.* Chicago, Aldine, 1965.
4. Cattell R: Factor analysis: An introduction to essentials. I. The purpose and underlying models, II. The role of factor analysis in research. *Biometrics* **21**: 190–215, 405–435, 1965.
5. McCloskey H, Schaar JH: Psychological dimensions of anomy. *Am. Soc. Rev.* **30**:14–40, 1965.
6. Nie NH, Hull CH, Jenkins JG, Steinbrenner K, Bent DH: *Statistical Package for the Social Sciences, second edition.* New York, McGraw-Hill, 1975.

Index